The Original Prescription

The Original Prescription

HOW THE LATEST SCIENTIFIC
DISCOVERIES CAN HELP YOU LEVERAGE
THE POWER OF LIFESTYLE MEDICINE

Thomas G. Guilliams Ph.D.
with Roni Enten M.Sc.

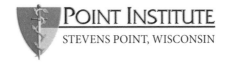

POINT INSTITUTE
STEVENS POINT, WISCONSIN

Disclaimer: The content and opinions in *The Original Prescription* are provided for educational and informational purposes only and are not intended as medical advice. This information should not be used to diagnose or treat any illness, metabolic disorder, disease, or health problem. Always consult your physician or healthcare provider before attempting to treat a serious or potentially serious condition.

Although the author and publisher have made every effort to ensure the accuracy and completeness of information contained in this book, we assume no responsibility for errors, inaccuracies, omissions, or any inconsistency herein. Any slighting of people, places, or organizations is unintentional.

Scripture quotations taken from the New American Standard Bible®.
Copyright © 1960, 1962, 1963, 1968, 1971, 1972, 1973, 1975, 1977, 1995 by The Lockman Foundation. Used by permission. (www.Lockman.org)

First printing 2012
ISBN: 978-0-9856158-4-0
LCCN: 2012940533

ATTENTION CORPORATIONS, UNIVERSITIES, COLLEGES, AND PROFESSIONAL ORGANIZATIONS: Quantity discounts are available on bulk purchases of this book for educational or gift purposes, or as premiums for increasing magazine subscriptions or renewals. Special books or book excerpts can also be created to fit specific needs. For information, please contact the Point Institute at www.pointinstitute.org.

DEDICATION

For Charlie, Dwight, and Nancy—

During the writing of this book I lost three dear friends. Each one endured their own health-related battles with dignity and with grace; each was taken before we wanted to let them go. They will be greatly missed.

Charlie Cutts was a dedicated servant of the Lord and a mentor to me since my youth. He and his wife, Shirley, took our family under their wing and were always a source of great joy. Charlie inspired my love of books but told me to wait until I was 40 before publishing my first. I only regret that he is not here to read it.

Dwight Pryor, founder of the Center for Judaic-Christian Studies, was the greatest teacher under whom I have had the pleasure to study. His ability to bring clarity to the most complex subjects was only exceeded by his love for and dedication to those he taught. His influence on my family and me is difficult to measure; may I be able to pass on just a portion of what he gave to me.

Nancy Dunahee arrived at Ortho Molecular Products just a few months before I was hired in 1996. In many ways, Nancy was the heart of Ortho. Whether it was her annual poem at the Christmas party or the little note to tell you she was praying for you, she always had her way of letting you know she was keeping her eye on things. Now she has a better view.

May their memory be for a blessing.

ACKNOWLEDGEMENTS

I WOULD LIKE TO personally acknowledge all those who have had a hand in making this book a reality. First to the dedicated researchers and clinicians I have met over the last two decades who have committed themselves to learning and teaching others about the wonderful healing capacity of the body, especially to all those who have lectured at IFM, ACAM, A4M, and the Medicines of the Earth conferences. The ideas in this book have been woven together from the many strands provided by their thoughtful presentations and discussions.

To all my friends and co-workers at Ortho Molecular Products—thank you for all your encouragement and your many persistent questions (especially all you sales reps); you made me dig deeper to find the answers. To the executive leadership team, for allowing me to dedicate the time to this project, and to Liz, who has been a steadfast and loyal assistant, allowing me to keep my sanity through the crazy schedule. To Roni, my research and writing assistant throughout this whole project, there is no telling when this project would have been accomplished without your help. To Nathan, for showing in figures what I am trying to explain in words. And to all those at About Books for helping to pull together this project in the crazy timeline I gave you.

Finally, I want to thank my family for their perseverance. My wife, Lori, and my children, Caleb, Naomi, Joshua, Katherine, Elisabeth, and Matthew; they have needed to do a few things without me during the writing of this book. They provide me with endless joy and have taught me the meaning of unconditional love. I promise I will wait a while for the next book project.

TABLE OF CONTENTS

PREFACE

THOSE WHO KNOW ME are well aware that I have spent over 16 years researching and developing evidence-based nutritional supplements (nutraceuticals) for use by clinicians and their patients. You might think it curious, then, that the first manuscript I decided to expand into a book is about lifestyle medicine. The reason is simple. I firmly believe that every therapy, including nutritional supplementation, must be rooted in the fundamental signaling pathways designed to keep us healthy. Those signals and that design are what this book is all about.

In many ways, I have been thinking about some of these ideas since my graduate school days, studying molecular immunology and debating the meaning of life with my fellow students. When you really begin to understand the elegant processes that drive the functions we call "life," you will just shake your head in amazement. My hope is that in my description of the simple complexity that converts our lifestyle decisions into health, you will first be amazed and then inspired to leverage these ideas to pursue your own optimal health.

The fundamental principles we outline here are not "new" per se; they are, after all, *The Original Prescription*. What is new is that our understanding of how and why these interventions work has been expanded with recent scientific research; and when we understand how something works, we are able to leverage its benefits. In this case, understanding the mechanisms behind lifestyle signals allows you to create a synergistic effect using multiple lifestyle intervention strategies. Knowing how these interventions work will also allow you to modify them to fit your unique health history and circumstance, and, because these concepts are fundamental principles, they won't become useless once the next health fad or research paper comes and goes. As an aside, my other great pursuit is the study of biblical history, language, culture and influence. I have included a few brief anecdotes from these pursuits, mostly in the form of footnotes, for your consideration as well.

It would have been easy in a book like this to point the finger of blame toward all those who have contributed to the poor lifestyles driving our healthcare crisis. The usual suspects of agribusiness, Big Pharma, insurance companies, fast-food chains, government regulation, FDA, poor parenting, and the like are easy targets. The fact is there is plenty of blame to be shared by all. Ultimately, most of the decisions that affect your health are yours to make. The principles outlined in this book have a powerful potential to turn your health around but are impotent if left neglected and untried. My hope is that you will, instead, choose to fulfill *The Original Prescription*.

T.G.G. —Jerusalem 2012

CHAPTER 1

The New Epidemic

"Truth is so obscure in these times,
and falsehood so established, that, unless
we love the truth, we cannot know it."

—Blaise Pascal (1623–1662)

IN APRIL OF 2009, two children in Southern California became ill with respiratory infections that, upon further diagnosis, were recognized as the first reported U.S. cases of a newly identified strain of H1N1 influenza virus (a.k.a. swine flu). There was no known connection between these two patients, nor had either been in contact with swine prior to their illness. A short while later, additional confirmed cases of H1N1, stemming from individuals traveling to Mexico, set off a series of steps that led the Centers for Disease Control and Prevention (CDC) to caution of a looming influenza epidemic; by June of that year, with the help of the World Health Organization, H1N1 was declared a global pandemic. For months, the evening newscasts were headlined by the number of confirmed H1N1 cases, the names of victims, and the status of the hoped-for vaccine. When the vaccine finally became available in October of 2009, demand quickly depleted all the available doses in many locations, and long lines formed anywhere claiming to have an available supply.

I recall writing an email editorial entitled "Pandemic or Pandemonium" just a few weeks after the CDC started its handwringing in early

May of 2009. I questioned whether the panic or the virus would be more potent, because early on it became fairly clear from the CDC's own data that the 2009 strain of H1N1 virus was less virulent than previous strains; or at least the outcomes were quite different than what the CDC had been projecting. You see, up to that point the CDC had been reporting that the *average* U.S. influenza-related death toll was approximately 36,000 deaths per year. However, the estimated number of influenza-related deaths in the U.S. between April 2009 and March 13, 2010, was 12,270 (various estimates ranged from 8,720 to 18,050), only 1/3 of the "average" annual flu-related deaths reported by the CDC up to that point. This discrepancy resulted in the CDC revising how it described its annual flu-related death rate, now reporting it as a 30-year range that is "from a low of about 3,300 deaths to a high of nearly 49,000."

Well, using either the older average (36,000 deaths per year) or the new range (3,300–49,000), it is clear that the fears of the 2009–10 influenza pandemic never materialized.[†] While much of the medical news was focused on H1N1, however, approximately 3,800 Americans were dying **each day** from heart disease, cancer, stroke, and diabetes. These causes alone totaled 1.38 million deaths in 2009 (more than half of all the recorded deaths). These represent numbers of epidemic proportion and constitute a true global pandemic. And yet getting the news anchors to report such numbers daily, or at all, is rare. What accounts for the disproportionate response to these two disease phenomena?

In past centuries, the global health crises have indeed been almost exclusively wide-spread, acute infectious and communicable diseases such as influenza, typhus, smallpox, cholera, and the plague. These devastating events, which sometimes resulted in the deaths of 30–40% of some national populations, left an indelible mark on these nations, and especially upon their public health apparatus. Focus was placed on quickly identifying infectious disease patterns, isolating infected individuals from the rest of the population, and aggressively inoculating populations in an attempt to immunize against the lethality of these diseases. At the same time, implementation of programs to improve hy-

---

† We certainly do not mean to minimize the tragedy of the lives lost to influenza or any other cause in making our broader point about the shift in disease patterns toward chronic metabolic diseases.

giene practices and access to clean food and water played a tremendous, some would say primary, role in limiting these epidemics.

During the centuries of revolving epidemics sweeping across the world, debates raged about the specific cause(s) of these diseases. To boil it down into the two prevailing camps, some thought that the causes were primarily external (filth, "miasmas," organisms, etc.) and others thought the causes were primarily internal (the physical, mental, or even spiritual status of the patient). In the end, external causes, or what we call the germ theory of disease, prevailed and have become the hallmark of infectious disease research ever since. Along with the works of Pasteur, Virchow, Lister, Fleming, and many others, Robert Koch is credited with defining the means to prove whether an organism is both necessary and sufficient to cause a specific disease. In a theory known as Koch's postulates, he outlined the required steps to isolate a specific organism from sick individuals, culture the organism, and then re-create the same illness/symptoms when that isolated organism was placed into another healthy individual. The very simplistic view of "cause and effect" demonstrated by Koch's postulates, based primarily upon the influence of external organisms, set in motion a monolithic and narrow definition of "disease" from which we are still trying to recover.

In the Western world at least, few truly devastating epidemics have occurred since the Spanish flu pandemic of 1918. In fact, the past century has seen a dramatic rearrangement of the causes of death in the West, including the U.S.: from classic infectious diseases such as influenza, pneumonia, and tuberculosis to chronic diseases such as heart disease, stroke, cancer, and diabetes. Unfortunately, the medical institutions we rely upon the most (as well as the media that communicates the news) are still better designed to identify and combat the infectious diseases of a century ago. Surveillance, quarantines, and mass vaccinations may be hallmarks of the diseases of decades ago, but they are hopelessly impotent to affect the metabolic diseases that are currently upon us. Certainly we don't want to lose our ability to detect and combat epidemic infectious diseases, but new strategies need to be developed to combat the new wave of chronic diseases that are plaguing us today.

Being able to recognize the changing patterns of epidemic trends is quite different than creating a solution that reverses these trends.

Because of the tremendous advances in our ability to identify and differentiate bacteria and viruses as the responsible infectious agents driving the epidemics of the recent past, the very concept of "disease" has been defined by those agents and the symptoms manifested by the infected: "Tuberculosis is caused by mycobacterium" or "Syphilis is caused by the spirochetal bacteria *Treponema pallidum*." In fact, the criteria used to identify what disease a patient had were (and still are) deciphered through a series of questions based primarily on the patient's symptoms: the presence or absence of a fever, a rash, a type of cough, diarrhea, or any number of other defining symptoms. By process of elimination, a diagnosis was made and a therapy prescribed. Invariably, this led to equating diseases with symptoms and eventually to the notion that treating symptoms was akin to treating (or even curing) diseases.

This simplistic "cause-and-effect" view of disease, however, has eluded us as we tackle the current swell of chronic diseases such as diabetes, heart disease, Alzheimer's disease and more. For instance, to say that lung cancer is caused by smoking cigarettes is still not the same as saying that the pox virus causes smallpox. It is possible, for instance, to develop lung cancer without ever being exposed to a cigarette; the same cannot be said of smallpox and the pox virus. There is no "Koch's postulate" for cancer, diabetes, obesity, or heart disease. In fact, what is becoming obvious as we understand more about the mechanisms driving this new wave of chronic diseases is that there is not a single specific cause of each of these conditions, unless you define the "cause" as the avoidance of behaviors known to prevent these diseases. Perhaps we should be spending less time looking into a microscope and more time looking into a mirror if we want to see the culprit of most of today's health problems.

So what then is driving these diseases if they are mostly preventable and not caused by infectious microbes?[†] Well, as we shall show, a combination of the lifestyle choices and environmental factors that characterize modern Western life appears to be the main culprit. What we

---

† That's not to say that microbes (bacteria, viruses, fungi) play no role in these disease phenomena at all; but it does appear that the classic cause-and-effect relationship between various microbes and chronic metabolic diseases, where an association might exist, is much more complex and highly dependent upon other factors in the host.

choose to eat and how much is just the tip of the iceberg. Not only have we radically altered our dietary patterns over the few past centuries, but physical activity, work patterns, social structure, leisure activity, stress, toxic burden, and sleep patterns have also dramatically changed. What we have deemed as the "progress" that currently defines civilized Western society may actually be slowly destroying human physiology.

The irony is that while the past century has been marked with an ever-increasing life expectancy in the U.S., the percent of the population suffering from debilitating chronic diseases is also growing. Perhaps life expectancy, often used as a generic measure of a population's health status, is a misleading indicator. This measurement reflects the average age at the time of death, so procedures or circumstances that reduce infant and childhood deaths will dramatically alter population life expectancy data. Furthermore, with the historical reductions in deaths caused by acute infectious diseases, our ability to prevent immediate deaths in individuals with severe life-threatening conditions is a hallmark of modern medicine. Whether from a heart attack, a car crash, or a gunshot wound, our emergency rooms are now able to save vastly more lives than they were a generation ago. Add to this organ transplants, artery bypass surgery, kidney dialysis, aggressive cancer drugs and surgery, along with other heroic (and expensive) measures, and the life expectancy has, until recently, continued to climb. But does this represent better health or better technology? What would our life expectancy numbers look like if we removed the artificial suspension of pharmaceutical drugs and heroic surgeries? Perhaps the overuse of simple statistical measurements, such as life expectancy, may actually have lulled us into a false sense of medical security.

But wait, wouldn't we just expect that since people are living longer, more chronic disease would be expected? Of course we would, but there is something else going on at the same time. At an alarmingly high rate, the age at which the first signs of many of these chronic diseases appear is getting lower and lower, countering the notion that the increase in chronic disease is only connected to age and increased life expectancy. The issue really boils down to health status. Preventing deaths by performing a quadruple bypass is not the same thing as improving someone's "health." Can we really compare the health of today's typical Medicare patient taking, on average, seven different pharmaceutical drugs with an individual of the same age 100 years ago? What is worse is that while the burden of chronic disease on the individual is clearly devastating, the burden on the healthcare system will eventually be overwhelming. Regardless of how we attempt to pay for the healthcare solutions of the future, we desperately need new approaches.

This year alone, millions of people will be diagnosed with diabetes or heart disease, while tens of millions more are right on the threshold. The current standard of care will dictate that each of these patients will receive one or more of the dozens of pharmaceutical agents approved for these conditions. At the same time, hundreds of billions of dollars will be spent by both industry and governments (through taxpayer-funded grants) looking to add one or two more drugs to the dozens or so we already have (likely replacing some that have been recalled)—and then more money will be raised, more grants will be written, and the process will begin all over again. The names of the drugs keep changing, but our solutions look much like they did a century ago.

Without question, the solution to our current wave of epidemic diseases must look very different than those of the recent past. After all, there is no equivalent to penicillin to make this go away. In fact, if the root causes of these new disease patterns are a result of our own lifestyle choices (individually and collectively), then the solution we seek must be based upon altering lifestyle choices. If 90% of the chronic metabolic diseases plaguing humankind today are preventable, why do we spend most of our money on solutions that avoid addressing the root cause? Science hasn't failed to give us the answers; scientists have just moved on to find answers that they think we will like better. Since we have failed to act by changing our lifestyle habits, we are paying them to discover the magic bullet, one that will allow us to somehow become healthy while ignoring our unhealthy habits.

The hypothesis in this book is simple. The current crisis that is soon to overwhelm healthcare systems around the globe is being driven by the accumulation of poor lifestyle decisions. While the harmful synergistic effects of these poor lifestyle decisions have taken decades to accumulate and overwhelm our buffer against chronic disease, our future is now partially controlled by the genetic modifications left behind by these poor decisions. We can stop and even reverse this chronic disease phenomenon (individually and globally) by understanding how our body turns lifestyle signals into health and applying a strategy that leverages the powerful synergy of good lifestyle decisions.

Our actions (or inactions) are the most powerful health-promoting tool we have. Our goal in this project is to reveal just how powerful lifestyle intervention really can be. We will be pulling back the curtain and peeking in on just how human physiology is carefully designed to maintain health and prevent disease if given the correct types and amounts of input. Using information from ancient sources up to the latest scientific discoveries in medicine, we hope to outline a new paradigm of thinking about health that explains how changes in our Western lifestyle patterns over the past few centuries have led to specific chronic disease patterns and how we can leverage the power of specific lifestyle changes to prevent and even reverse these disease processes. Recognizing the reality and severity of the current chronic disease burden, we also show how nutritional supplementation, alternative modalities, pharmaceuticals, and surgery can be incorporated within this paradigm.

The task ahead of us is quite challenging. First we will briefly discuss how obesity, one of the signs of Western success, is just the tip of an unhealthy iceberg, and then we'll move on to discuss how we got here in the first place. Understanding the recent past will open our eyes to just how dramatically things have changed. Then, since we spend quite a bit of time discussing a number of published scientific studies throughout the book, we will have a brief discussion about how we know what we know. Without bogging ourselves down in all the gory details, we will discuss the different ways that epidemiologists (those who study health and disease associated with populations) and sociologists (those who study human social structures) define the changes in human health and lifestyle over the past several centuries. Once we define the most prominent lifestyle alterations of the past, we will show how these changes participate in driving chronic disease. At that point, we will have laid the groundwork to introduce and explain the Lifestyle Synergy Model, a paradigm that explains how our bodies are designed to maintain wellness by converting signals from our lifestyle and creating the thing we call "health."

Once we have an understanding of the nuts and bolts of the Lifestyle Synergy Model, we begin to lay out the patterns and principles of a healthy lifestyle. First, we establish the seven different spheres or categories that define the synergistic approach to a healthy lifestyle (or a lifestyle intervention program). Then, we outline a series of principles to help implement the core ideas of each sphere. They are principles, not absolutes, so that you can adapt them and adjust them to new research and changing life situations. Ultimately these principles are the blueprint for health I call the *The Original Prescription* and, when implemented, have the power to turn your life and health around completely. Whether you are a clinician attempting to motivate patients to maintain their own health or a patient attempting to help yourself or a loved one regain health, these are the principles to live by.

Like the proverbial frog thrown into the pot of boiling water, the immediate crisis and fear of sudden death can generate immediate action, so it's no surprise that the threat of a potential flu pandemic quickly produces pandemonium. All the while, the frog sitting in the ever-warming water of poor lifestyle decisions doesn't realize that its demise will arrive without a moment's notice. Arming yourself with the knowledge of both the mechanisms and the principles of lifestyle medicine is the only way to build a healthy future, one that embraces and fulfills *The Original Prescription.*

CHAPTER 2

The Tip of the Iceberg

"Chronic diseases proceed from ourselves;
and although corpulency may be ranked amongst
the diseases arising from original imperfection in the
functions of some of the organs, yet it must be admitted
also to be most intimately connected with our habits of life."
—Thomas Sydenham (English physician; 1624–1689)

THIS IS NOT A book about obesity or, for that matter, a book about how to lose weight. That being said, one can hardly chronicle the plight of humans over the past few centuries without dealing with the global phenomenon of the obesity epidemic. As the proverbial "tip of the iceberg," we can easily measure the increased girth and weight of our neighbors and ourselves. And just like an iceberg, obesity's real danger lies beneath the surface—in the underlying physiological changes related to obesity, not to mention the growing burden this issue places upon our overextended healthcare system.

It is clear from almost every measurement that obesity (however we define it) increases the risk of nearly every chronic disease.[†] The most consistently studied conditions related to obesity are type 2 diabetes

---

† Obesity is medically defined as having a body mass index (BMI) greater than or equal to 30 kg/m², although risk is often related to visceral fat accumulation, which is measured by waist circumference or waist-to-hip ratio.

(which some researchers have likened the relationship to that of tobacco and lung cancer), cardiovascular disease, hypertension, stroke, and various forms of cancer. Together, obesity and diabetes are major causes of morbidity and mortality, with an estimated 300,000 U.S. adults dying each year of causes related to obesity.[1]

The magnitude of the obesity epidemic around the world has pushed weight-loss therapies to the forefront of modern life. In the U.S. alone, nearly 29% of men and 44% of women—an estimated 68 million adults—are trying to lose weight and spend over $30 billion a year in products and services related to weight loss.[3,4] For all of their investment, less than 20% of people attempting to lose weight are able to achieve and maintain a 10% reduction of weight over one year.[†] What's more, an increasing number of overweight and obese people have begun to turn to drastic surgeries for more rapid results. The annual rate of bariatric surgeries such as Roux-en-Y and lap-bands in the U.S. increased nearly six-fold between 1990 and 2000.[5] During the period between 2003 and 2008, the number of bariatric operations peaked at 135,985 cases and reached a plateau at 124,838 cases in 2008, revealing the gravity of this growing epidemic.[6] While it's true that many people are successful using these radical rescue interventions, it does not mean that we have made them fundamentally healthier as individuals. It pains me each time I hear of someone under the age of 20 who is convinced that permanently removing a portion of their GI tract is the only way to control their weight. How did we stray this far?

Obesity increases the risk of:[1]

- Coronary heart disease
- Type 2 diabetes
- Cancers (endometrial, breast, and colon)
- Hypertension
- Dyslipidemia
- Stroke
- Liver and gallbladder disease
- Sleep apnea and respiratory problems
- Osteoarthritis
- Gynecological problems (abnormal menses, infertility)[2]

---

† The emphasis on weight loss, sometimes by unhealthy means, is also partly driven by an unhealthy obsession with body image and thinness promulgated by Western fashion and commercial images. Unfortunately, this obsession with body image has confused the broader issues related to appropriate and healthy weight loss.

In one sense, chronic obesity is purely a human phenomenon. While some animals in the wild use fat mass to maintain body temperature (such as seals) or to survive hibernation (such as bears), there are no examples of chronically obese animals surviving comfortably in the wild. Now domesticated animals, they're quite a different story. So understanding obesity is much more than just explaining the physiology of adipose tissue, energy usage, and food composition; it really means understanding the human condition in a more profound way. In some ways, obesity is acting as a key physiological signal of the changing human condition over the past few centuries, telling us that these accumulated changes are overwhelming our body's ability to cope.

While history tells us that the *potential* for individual humans to become obese is very ancient, the notion that obesity can define a whole population is very new.[7] Stone-age figurines of obese individuals and even some depictions of obese individuals upon Egyptian stone reliefs imply that obesity was known and perhaps even venerated amongst some ancient peoples.[†] Ancient clinicians, however, were less impressed. Connections between diabetes and obesity are first hinted at in the Ebers papyrus of Egypt (1550 BC) referring to "*excessive urination*" and "*a medicine to drive away the passing of too much urine*."[8] The Greek historian Plutarch remarked that "*thin people are generally the healthiest; we should not therefore indulge our appetites with delicacies or high living, for fear of growing corpulent. ...The body is a ship which must not be overloaded.*"[‡] They could never have imagined the shipwreck we have today.

So how bad has the obesity epidemic become? In 2008, 1.5 billion adults across the world were classified as overweight (BMI>25); of these, 200 million men and nearly 300 million women were clinically obese, along with 43 million children under the age of 5. The amazing thing is that just 50 years ago, statistics on obesity prevalence did not even

---

† Some figurines of obese women are considered by some scholars to represent fertility goddesses, and often obese individuals are shown to be of royal or sacred status.

‡ The ancient Roman physician Galen recounted one of the earliest case studies of treatment for obesity this way: "*I reduced a huge fat fellow to a moderate size in a short time, by making him run every morning until he fell into a profuse sweat; I then had him rubbed hard, and put into a warm bath...Some hours after, I permitted him to eat freely of food, which afforded but little nourishment; and lastly, set him to some work.*"

exist.[9] In the early 1970s, only 14% of the U.S. population was classified as medically obese (BMI>30); today, obesity rates have more than doubled (in 2010, 12 states had an obesity prevalence over 30%, with Mississippi ranking the highest at 34%). The steady increase of individuals classified within the extremely obese (BMI >40) category is also an alarming new trend. To look at it another way, in the early 1960s the average American adult male weighed 168 pounds; today he weighs nearly 180 pounds. Over that same time period, the average female adult weight rose from 143 pounds to over 155 pounds.[10,11] These changes have become a noticeable problem over the past few decades, as many things we use on a daily basis were designed for a thinner population, such as airline seats, ambulance gurneys, hospital beds, folding chairs, and even coffins. Even drug doses were once considered normalized to a 150-pound adult—how "normal" is this today?

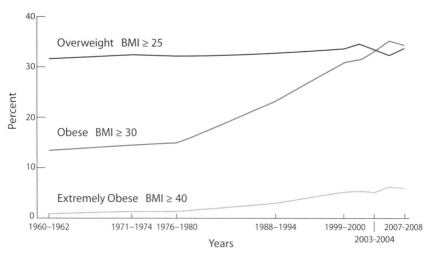

Figure 2.1 **Obesity Trends in the U.S. 1960–2008**

NOTE: Age-adjusted by the direct method to the year 2000 U.S. Census Bureau estimates, using the age groups 20–39, 40–59, and 60–74 years. Pregnant females were excluded. Overweight is defined as a body mass index (BMI) of 25 or greater but less than 30; obesity is a BMI greater than or equal to 30; extreme obesity is a BMI greater than or equal to 40.
SOURCE: CDC/INCHS, National Health Examination Survey cycle I (1960–1962); National Health and Nutrition Examination Survey I (1971–1974), II (1976–1980), and III (1988–1994), 1999–2000, 2001–2002, 2003–2004, 2005–2006, and 2007–2008.

The U.S. is not alone when it comes to obesity. Although nearly a third of the U.S. population today is considered obese,[12] in the U.K., the statistics are quite similar. In 2008, almost a quarter of the adults (24%

of men and 25% of women aged 16 or over) in England were classified as obese.[13] The story is similar in Australia, where over 17 million are overweight or obese.[14] But while the obesity epidemic has mostly afflicted Western countries, it is no longer restricted to industrialized societies alone. In fact, it is estimated that over 115 million people living within developing countries suffer from obesity-related problems, and these numbers are growing fast.[15] Many of these developing nations appear to be embracing Western lifestyle patterns at a rapid pace, resulting in equally rapid advances in obesity rates. Over the last few decades, profound changes have occurred in the quality, quantity, and sources of foods consumed in many developing countries. Combined with a decrease in overall physical activity among these same populations over the same time, these trends have led to an increase in the prevalence of obesity and diabetes and their related complications.[16]

Exporting a Lifestyle of Misery: Obesity and the Developing World

Obesity has long been perceived as a symbol of success or affluence, since socioeconomic status (SES) and place of residence have each been closely linked with the prevalence of obesity. In developing countries, a strong positive association is often seen between SES and obesity; lower SES individuals in these countries are more likely to engage in physical labor—and thus have a lower prevalence of obesity. Conversely, in those same developing nations, those with more resources and access to better nutrition, non-traditional foods, and labor-saving devices typically have a higher rate of obesity. In affluent nations like the U.S., the relationship between SES and obesity tends to be strong, but opposite (inverse) that of the developing nation. Food scarcity in industrialized nations is rare, and physical fitness often comes with greater costs, so we see higher obesity rates amongst those of lower SES in the U.S.[17] Since these phenomena cross national boundaries and ethnic and genetic barriers, this rapid spread to disadvantaged populations across the globe is one of the best pieces of evidence linking the role of lifestyle to the spread of obesity.

Over the last twenty years, obesity rates in developing countries have tripled where a Western lifestyle pattern has been adopted. In some cases, adopting a Western lifestyle pattern has literally devastated certain cultures from a health perspective. The highest rates of obesity in the world today are found among the Westernized peoples of the Pacific Islands, where rates of obesity are often over 70%.[†] In contrast, countries with strong cultures able to restrain the rate of Westernization have a much lower rate of obesity (India—just 0.5%; China, Japan, and the Philippines—3%; and Singapore—6%).[18] Consistent with this notion, surveys of seventy-five diverse communities in thirty-two different countries have shown that diabetes is rare when a traditional lifestyle has been preserved. This is often confirmed in studies showing that Arab, migrant Asian Indian, Chinese, and Hispanic communities in the U.S. that have undergone Westernization and urbanization are at much higher risk of diabetes than their counterparts who maintained traditional lifestyles.[19]

The classic example of this phenomenon is the Pima Indian population of North America, which has experienced one of the most dramatic rises in obesity levels of any population in the last century.[20] The rise in prevalence of obesity among the U.S. Pima Indians occurred during the post-World War II period, before which the population had limited contact with the Western world. Their traditional way of life was maintained until their water supply was diverted by farmers, facilitating their exposure to the Western lifestyle. Those born prior to this exposure to Western culture had a stable, healthy BMI throughout their whole lives; those born after WWII experienced a massive increase in BMI, which persisted throughout their entire lives.[21]

Compared to their genetically similar U.S. counterparts with the highest rates of diabetes in North America (38%), Pima Indians in Mexico, who have maintained a more traditional life in a rural environment, are substantially thinner and have one-fifth the prevalence of type 2 diabetes (7%). These data suggest that, even in a population with a high genetic susceptibility toward obesity and type 2 diabetes, these

---

† One of the highest is the American Samoan people—93.5% are overweight, while 80% of women and 69% of men are considered obese.

conditions are not inevitable and are preventable within an environment that promotes good lifestyle decisions. What is chilling is the swiftness of the changes in non-Western peoples adopting Western patterns of living. As we've shown, these changes in lifestyle have slowly accumulated over a few centuries in the West, leading to the steady increase in obesity and metabolic-related conditions, but when these accumulated changes have been transported, wholesale, into non-Western communities, these non-Western cultures are impacted in a single generation.

Obese Children: Our Future Health Burden

For me, the most alarming aspect of the obesity epidemic is the increased rate of childhood obesity over recent decades. Since 1980, obesity prevalence among children and adolescents has almost tripled, and obesity now affects 17% of all children and adolescents in the U.S. (12.5 million).[11]

The trend is similar in the U.K., where 16.8% of boys aged 2 to 15 and 15.2% of girls in the same age range were considered obese in 2008, as well as Australia, where 25.8% of boys and 24% of girls were either overweight or obese.[14] This trend is ominous for a number of reasons. For one, it is known that obese children are likely to experience much more severe obesity and the resulting consequences when they become adults.[13] Another is the fact that the offspring of obese individuals have a much higher risk of becoming obese, increasing with each succeeding generation. The future implications of these trends upon individuals and our healthcare system are unknown since such a drastic rise in childhood obesity is simply unprecedented.

Overall, the direct costs of obesity and physical inactivity accounted for approximately $147 billion of U.S. healthcare expenditures in 2008 alone, and if current trends continue, no healthcare system will be able to afford the increased financial burden.[22] It has been estimated that direct healthcare costs attributable to obesity and overweight conditions will more than double every decade, reaching $860-956 billion U.S. by 2030, or one in every six dollars spent on healthcare.[23] Unless the trends driving these patterns are reversed using methods similar to those we describe in the rest of this book, the consequences will be catastrophic.

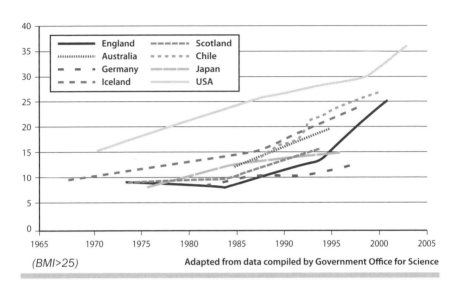

Figure 2.2 **Global Trend of Overweight Children by Percent**

(BMI>25)   **Adapted from data compiled by Government Office for Science**

A Way Forward

It doesn't require advanced scientific and medical acumen to realize that our health, as a population, is being devastated by the results of obesity. But diagnosing the symptom is not the same as understanding the root cause or devising a successful solution. Research companies will continue to tell us that there is a "cure" just around the corner, that a set of obesity genes will explain everything, or that a pharmaceutical solution is our only hope—maybe even as simple as something we can put in the water!

I think the answer is much different. Our physiology is designed to work when given a balanced set of inputs—what we might simply call a healthy lifestyle pattern. When we choose to avoid prudent lifestyle decisions and instead provide unhealthy patterns of signals, our bodies respond by tapping into available mechanisms to buffer the potential immediate threat posed by those unhealthy events. As we will show throughout the rest of this book, nearly every buffering mechanism used to help us prevent immediate health damage has an adverse effect upon the body's metabolic function, often causing it to use fat mass as a final buffering mechanism. Fat accumulation is the terminal and common pathway to most of the lifestyle stresses we encounter.

The current obesity epidemic, then, is a natural (and biologically expected) consequence of the accumulated changes and adaptations that our physiology has been making as we have altered nearly every part of our human existence over the past few centuries. It is the result of the power of Lifestyle Synergy, although as a negative force rather than a positive one.

If we are to use Lifestyle Synergy as a means to create health rather than disease, we need to understand not only how it works, but how to make it work for us. We need to look beyond the tip of the iceberg and see what lies beneath the surface.

CHAPTER 3

How We Got into This Mess in the First Place

"Those who cannot remember the past are condemned to repeat it."

—George Santayana (1863–1952)

IF HISTORY HAS TAUGHT us anything, it's that people pay little attention to history. Medicine, like most of the rest of life, is about what is new: a new drug, a new surgical procedure, a new diet, a new piece of exercise equipment, a new diagnostic test. Not only do we forget about what is "old," we cast it off as obsolete. Perhaps we have been just a bit too hasty. After all, obsolescence assumes that the new object performs all the functions of the old, with even more advantages to boot. Those of us living in the early 21st century can scarcely imagine functioning without the modern conveniences provided to us by the changing technology of the past two centuries. They are so integrated into our culture and experience, we hardly give a second thought to how many changes have actually occurred in that time span. Prior to 1800, technological advances were slow and often accessible only by the few elite who could afford such comforts. Today, most of these technologies are available to the majority of individuals within industrialized nations, and a vast number of people within developing nations as well. However, these advances in technology have not been without consequences. As we will chronicle in this chapter, the desire for more convenience has not been as benign as we would have thought.

A List of Some Advances since 1800

- Electric battery, electric motors
- The locomotive, the steamboat, the submarine
- Breech-loading guns (instead of muzzle-loading)
- The stethoscope
- Photography
- Internal combustion engine *(and everything that uses one)*
- The refrigerator
- The light bulb
- The sewing machine
- The telegraph and the telephone
- Artificial fertilizer
- Elevators and escalators
- Pasteurization
- The typewriter
- Margarine
- The vacuum cleaner
- The phonograph (record player)
- The fountain and ballpoint pen
- The kitchen stove
- Radio and television (and TV dinners)
- Plastic!
- The airplane
- The washing machine
- Microwave ovens
- Satellites
- Computers, the Internet, and every i-gadget

The opening chapter included a provocative assertion—that what we have deemed as the "progress" that currently defines civilized Western society may actually be slowly destroying human physiology. In order to convince you of that, a brief summary of how far our health-related lifestyles have changed is a necessary precursor to our later discussion about the mechanisms of lifestyle-related illnesses. I think you might agree after reading this chapter that many of the advances of the past several centuries have brought us a number of unintended and unforeseen medical consequences that new technologies are unlikely to repair.

We have all heard the adage "you are what you eat." And while this may not be physiologically accurate in all respects, our own health is greatly influenced by the 50 or so tons of food we consume in our lifetimes. Certainly what humans have been consuming over the past few generations has impacted what we have become from a medical perspective.

Until very recently, societal and cultural definitions were inextricably linked to the types of foods those societies and cultures consumed, which we typically referred to as their "traditional diet." These are still listed in the restaurant section of the phonebook (if you use such an archaic tome) or online by their various cuisines: Italian, Mexican, Chinese, Greek, and so on. So Americanized have these cuisines become that many have taken to adding "authentic" to their description in the hopes that we will think of them as untainted by our own food culture. But have you ever given much thought to how many changes have occurred in Western dietary patterns over the recent past and what the consequences of those changes have been? Let's briefly discuss the historical context of the major changes over the past few centuries—when "diet" became a four-letter word.

The Standard American Diet: S.A.D. Indeed

Since the second half of the twentieth century, the spread of the Westernized lifestyle across the globe has caused significant transformation in the dietary patterns of both industrialized and developing countries. These patterns of food consumption have been shown to be a key contributor to nearly every chronic disease, especially those related to cardiometabolic disease (heart disease, diabetes, etc.), that have now become global epidemics. Studies of pre-industrial and non-Western societies, such as parts of Asia and the Middle East, that were once burdened by under-nutrition now show growing numbers of obesity-related illnesses resulting from lifestyle factors. Most of these ills can be linked to the excess consumption of calories from animal fats, proteins, and sugar, along with a decreased consumption of vegetables, fruits, and complex carbohydrates—what is now often known as the Standard American Diet.[1] The Pima Indian example from chapter 2 is, regrettably, a classic illustration of this.

Dietary patterns and food selection are hallmarks of the historical study of human health and disease. Radical changes in eating habits have occurred in just the last century, creating a food environment that has been dramatically transformed over a relatively short period of time.[1] But according to the Institute of Medicine, since *"there has been no real change in the (human) gene pool in this period of increasing obesity, the root of the problem, must lie in the social and cultural forces that promote an energy-rich diet and a sedentary lifestyle."*[2] † Let's explore some of those social and cultural forces.

The Early American Diet

We recognize that the human diet, historically speaking, has forever been the result of an imperfect compromise between the struggle for survival and the provisions available within the local environment. Survival always meant having available food, water, and shelter. Eating foods in season before they spoiled was not some nutritional theory for our ancestors; it was a matter of life and death. The gathering of food was not only critical for survival; many of the daily tasks were designed around gathering, preparing, and consuming their daily bread. In modern times, this connection has deteriorated to the point where we can spend all day entertaining ourselves until deciding to "drive-thru" our favorite fast-food establishment and then speed away moments later with 2,500 calories that we can hastily consume while driving 70 miles per hour down a busy freeway. All of this can be completed in less time than it might have taken our forefathers just to gather enough wood for a cooking fire.

The first great food revolution came with the domestication of plants and animals. The advent of agriculture across the world shifted the human diet from fruits, roots, and vegetables gathered from the local surroundings; animal foods derived from wild (hunted) animals;[3] and a few delicacies like honey (one of the few concentrated sugars available on a seasonal basis)[3] toward a host of novel foods. In the Americas, corn, beans, and squash were among the earliest crops, and domesticated animals were introduced soon after. Cereal grains, dairy, sugars, oils, fatty meats, and salt followed in the fertile and abundant land.

---

† While we generally agree with this IOM statement, epigenetic changes discussed in a later chapter likely have a profound effect on how food and other lifestyle activities drive the disease mechanism and are an important part of the Lifestyle Synergy Model discussed in chapter 5 and beyond.

The arrival of European agricultural and food practices in America shaped local food preferences. The types of foods consumed reflected regional differences, but the common cooking habits and food preparation methods stayed true to Anglo-Saxon culinary traditions across the country.[4] In New England, the population enjoyed bread, bacon, and beans with root vegetables as staple foods, while in the South, pork and corn were the main staples.[4] Despite the abundance of food throughout most of the country, much of the American population suffered from malnutrition due to a lack in both quality and variety. In the winter, Nnorthern diets consisted mostly of potatoes, cabbage and turnips, pickled condiments, and watered-down milk colored with chalk, while farmers in the South lived mostly on bacon, corn pone, and coffee with molasses.[4] By the 1870s, canned fish, fruit, vegetables, and milk became more widely available and supplemented the simpler diets that were lacking in these food groups.

Among more affluent Americans, meats and starches were favored as main dishes at mealtime along with vegetables, typically boiled over several hours, which were served as side dishes. Apples were a mainstay of the diet and were often eaten as a key source of dietary fiber. Foods fried in butter and lard were very popular, and the growing national sweet tooth was satiated with various puddings, sweet condiments, and sauces. The theme of the American diet even then was to indulge in the nation's great abundance whenever possible at breakfast, lunch, and dinner.[4] At the time, however, most Americans labored long enough to burn even this high number of calories.

> *"There was oatmeal with plenty of thick cream and maple sugar. There were fried potatoes, and the golden buckwheat cakes, as many as Almanzo wanted to eat, with sausages and gravy or with butter and maple syrup. There were preserves and jams and jellies and doughnuts. But best of all Almanzo liked the spicy apple pie, with its thick crust, rich juice and its crumbly crust. He ate two big wedges of the pie."*
>
> —from *Farmer Boy* by Laura Ingalls Wilder[5]

Pre-industrial Food and Preparation Methods

Up until about 1830, before canning became widely available, common food preservation methods included salting, spicing, smoking, pickling, and drying, with little need for refrigeration of foods such as meat, fish, milk, fruits, and vegetables.[6] Consumer demand for an abundance of fresh produce grew as the rapid expansion of cities was combined with a general improvement in the economic status. Demands to increase the distance that food could be transported, from producer to consumer, improved the diversity of the common diet and allowed for food and nutrient combinations not possible in previous generations.

By the 1920s, the household refrigerator became available and profoundly altered the American diet, becoming an essential component of the American kitchen and permanently expanding the available food choices. While families were once dependent on ice deliveries to keep food fresh and readily available for meal preparation, perishable foods such as meat, dairy, and produce could now be stored more conveniently without spoiling. By 1931, over one million refrigerators had been manufactured in the U.S.; by 1937 that number had reached almost six million.

Since dairy products could now be kept fresh in the home, the demand for them grew at a quick pace. Dairy farming soon expanded from the small backyard herd to larger industrial farms, providing people all over the country with fresh milk, butter, and cream on a regular basis. The growing scale of production within the dairy industry spurred new needs in both processing and purity, which led to the implementation of pasteurization, the heating of milk to kill off pathogens and natural enzymes that contribute to spoilage, and homogenization practices. Commercial pasteurization of milk reached the U.S. in the early 1900s and reduced mortality in infants from milk-borne illness; homogenization delayed the separation of cream and allowed the milk of many dairy cows to be blended into one uniform flavor and texture.[7] With the growing demand for dairy, the average American cow had been transformed rapidly into a food industry.

Along with dairy, beef—a longtime staple in the American diet—became more widely available with the expansion of cattle lands westward. Before 1850, virtually all cattle in the U.S. were free-range or pasture-fed and typically slaughtered at 4-5 years of age.[3] With the lowering of prices due to expansion of cattle ranches and the increasing negative view of pork as unwholesome and difficult to digest, beef grew in popularity.[4] By 1885, cattle were fattened rapidly in feedlots on a new source of nourishment—corn, which changed the nutritional make-up of American beef, making it possible to ready a fattened steer for slaughter, marbled to perfection, in just 24 months.[3]

Growing stocks of poultry offered yet another main source of protein that was now readily available to families, and the building and expansion of railroads in the 1880s helped to effectively transport all of these major staples across the country.[4] Even lettuce, which was once limited to the wealthy because of its fragility, experienced a jump in consumption in 1903 with the development of the iceberg variety, chosen for its hardy structure and "shelf life," bringing this vegetable into refrigerators across America.[4]

The advent of the breakfast cereal was also pivotal in changing the American diet. Cereal was quicker to prepare than meat-based breakfasts, and its clean packaging served the growing demand for "germ-free" food; quick-to-fix cereal soon replaced the tradition of the large American breakfast for many, and catchy names attested to the clever advertising and promotion that were developing within the industry. Other examples of popular packaged food products of the day included boxed crackers, Heinz condiments (which also promised to lessen the burden on housewives to prepare sauces and dips from scratch), and canned soups. As the industry expanded, the selection of processed foods followed suit, meeting the growing demands of Americans for purity, variety, and convenience.

The American Diet: An Industrial Solution

The industrialization of agriculture and the American diet meant that food scarcity and lack of selection became a thing of the past, allowing opportunities for new food processing procedures as well as novel food products. From the pre-industrial era through the 1960s, food gathering and preparation took up most of a woman's days, and the bulk of food preparation was done for consumption at home.[4] Even in 1965, married women who didn't work outside the home still spent over two hours per day cooking and cleaning up from family meals. By the mid-90s, these tasks consumed less than half that time. It appears that each passing generation is investing less and less time with their food, leaving it up to others to package and prepare their very sustenance.

Technological innovations, such as vacuum packing, deep freezing, artificial flavors, and artificial preservatives, allowed manufacturers to cook food from a central location and ship it to consumers for faster and more convenient consumption. The switch from individual to mass preparation lowered the time required, as well as the price of food consumption, and led to the increased quantity and variety of foods consumed.[8] More food abundance and availability inevitably led to increases in the average Americans' dietary intake. Energy intake per capita over just the last half century increased from 1,900 calories in the late 1950s to a whopping 2,661 calories in 2008, with most of this increase occurring between 1970 and today.[9] Portion sizes have also continued to grow over time, far exceeding those consumed historically. For instance, the average fast-food hamburger grew in size from one ounce in 1957 to up to six ounces in 1997. Not surprisingly, the evidence shows that when larger portion sizes are provided, more food is eaten.[10]

The New Western Staples: Refined Flour, Sugar, and Vegetable Oil

White Flour

While flour, oil, and sugar were always part of the American diet, the proportion and nutritional content of these food staples changed even more profoundly with the introduction of food-processing procedures.[3] Prior to the industrial revolution, cereals were ground with stone milling tools, and flours contained the entire contents of the grain, including the germ, bran, and endosperm.[3] Beginning in the 1840s, new flour milling processes were introduced, and white flour, stripped of its germ and bran components, became a staple in the American diet. At the time, the removal of the germ and bran allowed for longer storage of flour, making it easier to produce all sorts of breads and pastry.

Ironically, white flour was considered by some to be "healthier" because it was less likely to spoil. Later, when it was realized that vital nutrients were lost in the refinement process, fortification of iron, thiamin, riboflavin, niacin, and folic acid was introduced, and the enrichment of white flour continues to this day. In fact, the easy access to prepared grains in the form of enriched white flour has contributed to the single greatest increase in calories since the 1950s, followed closely by sugar.[9] On average, Americans today consume 8.1 ounce equivalents of grains per day, 7.2 ounces of which come from refined grains.[9] In 2000, Americans consumed an average of 200 pounds of flour and cereal products per year, compared to just 135 in the early 1970s.[11]

Sugar

In the mid-19th century, Americans were already consuming the most sugar in the world, and by 1970, the consumption of refined sugars per capita in the U.S. reached over 120 pounds per person every year. In 2000, that number had increased to over 150 pounds. Today, approximately 37% of added sugars consumed by Americans comes from sweetened carbonated beverages, followed by candy, cakes, cookies, and pies.[9]

The link between our current crisis of metabolic diseases and sugar consumption includes an interesting twist—the intake of significant calories through sugar-sweetened beverages. The consumption of sweetened carbonated beverages, which first became popular in the late 1800s, has spiked dramatically in the last fifty years. In 1942, the annual production of carbonated soft drinks in the U.S. was the equivalent of sixty 12-ounce servings per person, an average of just over one serving/week.[12] In 1957, most soft drinks were served as 8-ounce bottles, but that ballooned to 32- and even 64-ounce containers by 1997.[13] Between 1942 and 2005, production of soft drinks increased ten-fold, although the increase in the population only just doubled.[12] Soft drink consumption increased especially among adolescents. In the fifteen years between 1979 and 1994, adolescent boys and girls increased their average daily consumption of soft drinks by 74% and 65%, respectively, while milk consumption decreased among these groups over this period.[14] Today, Americans consume twice as many sweetened carbonated beverages as they did 25 years ago, adding an estimated 411 calories daily from these beverages at a cost of over $54 billion a year.[9,15] While some feel protected by consuming diet versions of these soft drinks, artificial sweeteners still promote the need for sweetened beverages and have not shown themselves to be a healthy alternative. In fact, consumption of diet soft drinks has been linked to increased risk of metabolic syndrome, type 2 diabetes, and stroke.[16,17]

Vegetable Oil

In the past five decades, we have seen a major shift in the fats and oils used in cooking. Prior to that time, butter and lard were the preferred products; since then, however, we have undergone a bit of a revolution due to the production and processing of fats derived from oily seeds (soybean, corn, sunflower, safflower, rapeseed, etc.). Technological breakthroughs in the development of high-yield oilseeds, combined with the process of refining high-quality vegetable oils, greatly reduced the cost of baking and frying with fats and allowed for the availability of new products such as margarines, salad dressings, spreads, and cooking oils, all of which were consumed more widely and on a more regular basis.[18] Similar to the growth in refined flour and sugar, during the ninety years from 1909 to 1999, per capita consumption of salad and cooking oils jumped 130%, shortening consumption grew 136%, and margarine consumption increased 410%, all significant changes in both quantitative and qualitative aspects of fat intake.[3]

Many people consider the transition away from saturated fats such as butter and lard toward polyunsaturated seed oils as a positive food trend, and in some ways they are correct. That this trend has not produced the sort of benefit one would have predicted, I believe, is due to four factors, which we will only have time to mention briefly here.

The first is simply that we are consuming more fat calories; polyunsaturated fats often serve as an addition to, rather than a replacement for, saturated fat calories. The second is that the availability of abundant cheap liquid oils has made the deep-frying of food ubiquitous in the U.S., reducing the nutritional benefit of nearly everything prepared in this manner. On a related note, the heating and modification of polyunsaturated fatty acids from seed oils (especially in prepared foods) to create partially hydrogenated oils introduced a new fatty acid structure known as "trans-fatty acids," compounds now limited by FDA within foods because of their known harm to our health but for years touted as preferential to the saturated fats they replaced. Finally, an effect that was unforeseen with the mass introduction of seed oils was the increased shift in human omega-6 versus omega-3 fatty acid intake. This shift toward higher levels of omega-6 fatty acids is known to promote a higher inflammatory burden, contributing to the process of chronic disease.[19]

Disappearance of the Family Meal

The changes in the Western dietary pattern are not limited to food and food processing methods alone; they have also been greatly impacted by the changes in the environment in which those foods are consumed. The traditional pattern of families eating together at the kitchen table is in decline, and, unfortunately, statistics show Americans are eating more and more of their meals away from the kitchen table. As one might imagine, foods consumed at family meals have been shown to be generally more nutritious, particularly for children and adolescents. Studies suggest that those eating dinner at a family meal had higher consumption of fruits and vegetables, fiber, folate, calcium, iron, and vitamins B-6, B-12, C, and E, and lower consumption of saturated and trans-fatty acids, soda, and fried foods.[13,20]

By 1995, 57% of Americans consumed at least one food item away from home on any given day, up from 43% in 1978.[21] Today, children consume a quarter of their meals away from the family table, and the numbers increase as they get older (18% for preschoolers, 26% for school-age children, and 30% for adolescents); fast-food restaurants account for more than 50% of those meals eaten outside the home.[13,22] The broader psychosocial benefits of regular family meals are difficult to measure but have been related to better social adjustment and school grades in children and youth, as well as reduced likelihood of smoking, drinking, and drug use in later adolescence.[23]

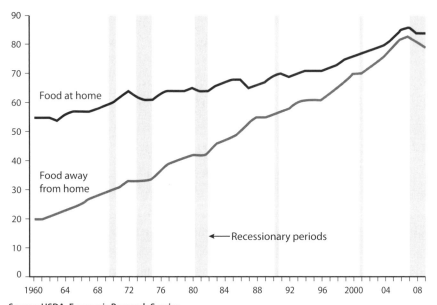

Figure 3.1 **Food Expenditures Home and Away**

Source: USDA, Economic Research Service.
Recessionary periods determined by National Bureau of Economic Research.

Note that while the amount spent on food at home has gone up only 50% in the past 50 years, food away from home has increased by 300%!

The decreased time spent preparing and eating family meals at home is partially due to busy schedules; over 1/3 of U.S. parents say they eat takeout food regularly, and 1/5 of all meals are consumed in a car, with over 12% of calories for adults coming from fast food.[24,25] Ironically, the advent of all the labor-saving devices we have created over the past few centuries seems to have decreased, rather than increased, our ability to prepare and consume foods.[26]

Even meals eaten at home very often are consumed away from the family meal setting. One of the hallmarks of this trend was the rise of the TV dinner in 1954, which appealed to a widespread desire to prepare meals at home in less time.[25] The microwave oven, which made TV dinners even more convenient, also reduced the need to plan for meals.[25] Developed in the 1940s, microwave ovens became more widely available in the 1970s. According to the Energy Information Administration, only 8% of American households had microwave ovens in 1978, but by 1999, 83% did.[8] A new definition of "cooking" emerged as people were now able to "nuke" food from the freezer to the table in just two minutes.

Snack Attack

These changes in the American mealtime traditions have also encouraged the popularization of snacks. A snack is technically any food consumed between meals, using the traditional definitions of breakfast, lunch, and dinner.[†] And while snacks can be consumed as an appropriate response to hunger, they are often eaten by habit, independent of hunger signals. Studies have shown that much of the increase in calories in the average American diet is from snacks and that the growth in overall caloric intake is due to a greater frequency of eating rather than simply eating more at any one sitting. Between 1977 and 1978, only about 28% of people reported eating two or more snacks per day, but 45% reported two or more snacks from 1994 to1996, with the average number of snacks per day increasing by 60% during the intervening period. In addition, the percentage of students eating snacks increased from 60% in 1977–1978 to 75% in 1994–1996. Nearly all children reported eating at least one snack per day, and 36% of children consumed at least four or more different daily snacks. Other studies of adolescents show similar dietary patterns; snacking is clearly a main contributor to obesity among youth and adults.[13]

Unintended Consequences of Food Miles

Studies estimate that processed foods in the United States travel over 1300 miles before being consumed, while some fruits and vegetables often log over 1500 miles. This may be great when I am looking for

---

† There is a debate today about the role of the traditional three-meal-per-day approach. Many consider it better to consume fewer small meals/snacks throughout the day to maintain metabolic balance and steady glucose. We are not debating the pros and cons of that approach here. Historical evidence suggests that increased snacking, for the majority of Americans, contributes additional calories to the three-meal-per-day approach.

a pineapple or a mango in central Wisconsin, but what are the implications of this phenomenon?

The fresh and local markets that still thrive in the developing world have all but disappeared as the major source of food supply in the West. Instead, they have been replaced by multinational or regional chains of large supermarkets.[27] Another example from the Midwest shows the trend well; in 1870, 100% of the apples consumed in Iowa were produced in Iowa, but in 1999, Iowa farmers grew only 15% of the apples eaten in the state.[28] To accommodate these food miles, produce must be picked early and ripened in a controlled fashion, at the expense of both freshness and nutrient content. The price of produce is therefore tied to rising fuel prices. Between 1985 and 2000, fruits and vegetables led all other food categories in increased retail price. The high price of produce contributes to the perception that eating "healthy" is less affordable than eating convenience-based foods.

No doubt there are many other changes to our food habits that we could mention, but as you can see from this brief stroll through human food history, the changes that have occurred just in the past 200 years are astounding.[4,8] And while it is tempting to pin all our health issues upon these changes alone, a number of other radical alterations in human behavior occurred at the very same time—we will explore some of those next.

Striving to Strive Less

Over the past two centuries, the drop in the level of human physical activity in the West has sparked a seismic shift in lifestyle that has fundamentally impacted the health of people across the globe. The Western lifestyle, built upon and characterized by physical labor, has become largely sedentary and, together with dramatic changes in diet, is now one of the most significant contributors to the major chronic diseases of today.

Today's modern, Westernized lifestyle is the result of a process of industrialization that gradually altered the daily lives of people across the globe over the last 200 years. Today, most of our domestic and daily tasks require little of the physical effort they once did, since almost all of these tasks have become completely automated. Along with that automation, similar technological advancements have occurred in the world of leisure-time activity, centered primarily on the TV and the computer.

Prior to industrialization, the function and survival of the family unit were the driving forces behind a lifestyle characterized by high levels of physical activity. Families, which were both larger in size and rural in setting, were for the most part self-sustaining, producing much of what they needed for support and trade in the market.[29] Pre-industrial families, including both adults and children, spent their time almost entirely on household tasks and chores, with much less time available for leisure activities. In today's post-industrial society, however, the household is no longer the center of production; families are located in more urban settings, and their basic function and tasks have changed significantly.

Changes in the home were mirrored in many ways by changes in industry. Hand power was replaced by steam and electric power; coal and wood were replaced with gas and oil as fuels for cooking. Pumping water was no longer required when running water became readily available, and washing machines replaced basins of boiling water and wash boards; all were major advances in technology that allowed people to work less and have more time for leisure. Domestic mechanization has notably shifted the work practices of women in particular, as many of the labor-saving devices now used in homes replace or simplify tasks done predominantly by women.[30]

Indeed, there is little question that wide-scale automation has substantially impacted the energy expenditure of people living a Westernized lifestyle. Research has shown that sales of domestic labor-saving devices and vehicles are correlated with obesity prevalence rates, even where trends in energy and fat intake do not appear to have changed.[31-35] In one study, modern actors mimicking the lifestyle of 19th-century "Old Sydney Town" (Australia) recorded 60% higher physical activity levels compared to controls living a modern life.[36] Between 1950 and 2000 alone, the prevalence of sedentary occupations in the U.S. rose from 23% to 41%.[38] Today, in stark contrast with pre-industrial Americans, U.S. children and adults spend approximately 55% of their waking hours, or 7.7 hours/day, in behaviors that result in very low levels of energy expenditure. Older adolescents (ages 16–19 years) and older adults (ages 60–85 years) spend nearly 60% of their time, or more than eight hours per day, in sedentary behaviors, and children aged 6–11 years spend six hours per day sedentary.[39]

Heating a Rural Home in 1800

- Find deadfall or cut down tree(s)
- Cut trees into manageable sizes using axe or hand saw
- Split wood if necessary
- Haul wood to dry storage location and stack
- Regularly haul dry wood into home
- Start/maintain fire
- Regularly remove ashes
- Repeat each step regularly

Washing Clothes in a Rural Home in 1800

- Gather wood for fire
- Haul water from pump or creek
- Start fire under vessel of water
- Hand-wash clothes with soap (likely also homemade)
- Rinse clothes and hang to dry

Heating an Urban Home in 2010

- Set or program thermostat once
- Authorize automatic payments online

Washing Clothes in an Urban Home in 2010

- Place clothes in washing machine with detergent; press button
- Move clothes to dryer; press button

Television: Leisure Time Extraordinaire

Few things define Westernization like the television. Today, 99% of American households have at least one television set, and the majority has more than one.[40,41] TV viewing far exceeds the time spent in any other leisure activity and represents the principal sedentary behavior in the U.S. In fact, the largest single replacement for the time made available by reduced housework is television viewing. Today, computers, personal electronic devices, and video games come in a close second to TV in terms of accumulated sedentary time.

Most concerning are the statistics measuring the time children spend watching television. In the United States, children watch an average of three to four hours of television per day, which means that by high school graduation, average Americans will have spent more time watching television than they have in the classroom.[42]

Since the first research conducted on the subject more than two decades ago, dozens of studies have established and confirmed the connection between the time spent watching TV and obesity rates in adults and children.[43] The prevalence of obesity is over four times greater among individuals who watch twenty-one or more hours of TV per week compared to those who watch fewer than seven hours per week.[1] In 1985, researchers showed that for each additional hour spent watching TV, prevalence of obesity increased by 2% among a large sample of children.[43,44]

When we combine the changes of the past centuries—the decreased labor involved in regular domestic life, the dramatic increase in sedentary or mostly sedentary jobs, and the hours spent in sedentary leisure activities—it is easy to see that we are in a heap of trouble.[45] † These behavior changes have become substantial contributors to the morbidity and mortality of chronic diseases in the U.S. Today, sedentary lifestyle ranks only behind cigarette smoking and obesity as the key contributor to deaths from nine major chronic diseases, including coronary heart disease, stroke, diabetes, and colorectal cancer. The couch potato lifestyle was estimated to account for approximately 23% of all deaths from these causes.

Too Stressed to Sleep

The last two trends we want to explore before moving on are related to one another. One is the increased level of stress upon the human condition, and the other is the decreasing amount of sleep in modern

---

† I have become acutely aware of this in the past several years as my own job requires me to spend hours reading studies, writing reports, and responding to an endless stream of emails— mostly while seated. I have yet to master the standing or treadmill desk concept.

industrial life; the latter is a bit more measurable than the former. For instance, the average duration of sleep among U.S. citizens has been dropping for more than a generation. In 1959, the median sleep duration in adults aged 40–79 years was eight hours per night, with only 15% reporting less than seven hours per night; by 2002, the median sleep duration had dropped to seven hours, with more than 33% reporting fewer than seven hours of sleep.[46,47]

So why exactly have we been losing sleep over the last centuries? One could surmise that with all the extra time saved throughout the day, we would have more time to sleep rather than less. But it simply isn't so. With the advent of electric lights, we were no longer compelled to sleep when the sun went down or required to fumble with the limited light produced by candles or lanterns, so we extended our days with both work and play—shortening the length of time we spent sleeping. Entertainment, especially in the form of television watching, is partly to blame, as studies have shown a clear relationship between short sleep duration and increased hours spent watching TV.[48] Since a significant amount of television viewing is carried out at or near bedtime, sleep is necessarily delayed and often even prevented.[49]

Recent research has clearly shown that poor sleep patterns, especially short sleep duration, play a significant role in the modern obesity pandemic, with its related increased risk for diabetes and heart disease.[†] According to recent statistics, 50–70 million Americans suffer from some sort of insomnia, and in 2010, up to 10% of Americans were taking prescription sleeping medication. This is disturbing for a number of reasons, not the least of which is that recent data suggest that individuals taking sleeping pills are up to three times more likely to die early than those who have never used these medications.[50] This means that early death is in some manner attributed to sleep disorders, sleeping pills, or another root cause of sleeping disturbances. Likely all three contribute a portion of the risk.

Finally, there is stress. Few things define modern life like this one single word. As we will discuss more thoroughly in chapter 10, stress plays a major role in the pathophysiology of nearly all chronic disease,

---

† We will explore many more details on the role of sleep in chapter 11, where we examine the emerging science of chronobiology.

but since stress as a medical concept is difficult to measure, we can only say what few would dispute: stress levels have been growing more and more as the metabolic burden has increased. In some ways, stress is both a contributor to and a product of all of these changes. Our diet, our physical inactivity, our growing inflammatory burden, our poor sleep habits, our changes in family dynamics and relationships, our changing work schedules, our growing burden of electronic gadgetry—all contribute to our stress, which itself drives more metabolic-related disease.

The massive volume of change upon the human physiology over the past century, only partly described in this chapter, is clearly more than we, or our healthcare system, can handle. Many of the signals to which humans were once accustomed, the ones keeping us healthy, are absent, having been replaced by a new set of signals that work against our health. These poor signals work together to produce a powerful negative synergistic influence on all systems of the body. They reinforce and build off one another, destroying individuals, families, communities, and nations. Identifying the myriad of signals that are hidden in these lifestyle changes and understanding how they influence our health are the first steps in leveraging them to our advantage. The same powerful effects are also available when we turn the equation around—when we choose to make good lifestyle decisions. This is ultimately the power of the Lifestyle Synergy Model.

CHAPTER 4

How We Know
What We Know

"If we knew what it was we were doing,
it would not be called research, would it?"

—Albert Einstein (1879-1955)

BEFORE WE MOVE FURTHER into what defines the Lifestyle Synergy Model and ways to leverage these ideas to reverse the current disease crisis, we need to take a brief detour. In some ways, this might be the most important chapter of this whole book because it helps explain how to understand the results derived from scientific research, something that will help you evaluate any future information related to your health. In the time it took to write this book, tens of thousands of research articles were published and thousands of ground-breaking studies were announced at symposia throughout the world, many of which have altered the way we understand medicine and human disease. If you are serious about healthcare solutions, as the one on either the giving or the receiving end, then you must understand how scientific information is turned into therapeutic recommendations. In other words, you must understand how we know what we know.

As someone who spends a significant amount of time attempting to stay on top of the vast amount of medical and scientific research, I understand why it is so difficult to make sense of it all. And since I speak regularly with clinicians, I know this is especially true for both them and their patients. Should we be consuming fewer fats or fewer carbs? Should we be recommending regular mammograms or avoiding them altogether? Which women will benefit from hormone replacement therapy and which women will be harmed? Would the use of bio-identical hormones instead of pharmaceutical hormones change the risk/benefit equation? How many glasses of water should we drink every day? Should we recommend sun exposure in order to increase vitamin D or avoid the sun and use sunscreen to prevent UV-induced harm? Can we prove that organic foods are better than conventionally-grown foods? And so on and so forth.

If you have been attempting to follow the published medical literature and the ensuing media coverage, you could probably add a few dozen more questions to the list. The confusion created in the wake of all these reports has left many frustrated and skeptical. Unfortunately, this has served as an excuse for many individuals to do nothing about their unhealthy lifestyle, ignoring the obvious signs of chronic disease progression. Furthermore, clinicians often don't know which way to turn. Should they stick with the guidelines that might be ten or more years old? Or should they attempt to follow something new (and controversial) they just heard at a meeting? Perhaps they should wait to see what will be reimbursed by the insurance provider of the patient before recommending anything?

What we hope to do in this chapter is help explain why scientific and medical research results can be so confusing and help navigate through the many types of studies being published. I often say that science is a double-edged sword; the intention is to answer a question, but often the result merely introduces a new set of questions. Just when we think we have "figured it out," we discover something that turns everything we have known on its head. What seemed obvious and proven to one generation is debunked by the next, often to be revived by future generations that end up proving the original thinkers right after all. We can't deal with every nuance related to research here, of course, but a brief stroll through the neighborhood will help give perspective to the concepts and the research cited throughout the chapters ahead.

What Type of Study Is It?

Smoking cigarettes causes cancer. There are few people nowadays who would generally dispute this statement; but is this statement scientifically true? After all, we have all met smokers who will tell us of someone who smoked their whole lives and remained cancer-free until the end. The FDA claims that 90% of lung cancer deaths in men (80% in women) are due to cigarette smoking, yet 90% of men who smoke do not get cancer. So while the FDA requires a package of cigarettes to warn "Smoking Cigarettes Causes Cancer," this statement really means "Smoking cigarettes will greatly increase your risk for cancer; nine out of ten lung cancer deaths occur in smokers."

Why is this nuance important? While the smoking/cancer connection has ceased to be controversial, replace the conversation with something like drinking coffee, eating eggs, consuming soy, or using hormone replacement therapy or antibiotics, and now the nuances become very important. Studies over the past decade seem to alternate between beneficial effects and harmful effects for most of these substances. This is why it is so important to ask, "What type of study was this?" Is it a human study, an animal study, or a cell-culture-based study? Are these results based on large populations, or is this a defined group of individuals in a controlled clinical trial? Understanding the basic types of scientific and medical research can be very helpful when attempting to make sense of the information being presented.

Types of Medical Research

Basic Science	This is a broad category of research which includes biochemistry, molecular biology and the mechanisms of compounds upon cells and tissues outside of the organism. *In vitro* research falls into this category and might involve human, animal or bacterial cells.
Animal Studies	As the name implies, this includes research done using animals as subjects. In many cases there are animal models which mimic the responses of specific human diseases.

(continued)

Human Studies

Case-Studies and Case-Series	These are reports where clinicians write up the description of a unique patient case, or a series of patient cases which tell a particular story. This is highly specialized anecdotal information; often to tell of a rare disorder, a diagnostic anomaly or an unusual response to treatment.

Observational Studies (Epidemiology)

Case-Control	This study selects cases (those with a disease) and controls (individuals with similar traits but without the disease) and attempts to discover differences in habits or events of these individuals. (retrospective)
Follow-up Design	This type of study takes a group (cohort) of "healthy" individuals, measures a number of baseline characteristics and follows them over time for disease outcomes. (prospective, but non-interventional)
Cross-Sectional	Here we simply take a cross-section of people (all patients in a specific clinic or town) and divide them based on a specific criteria and risk factors. (neither prospective nor retrospective)

Experimental Studies (Clinical Trials)

Pre-Clinical Studies	These types of studies are used in very small groups of patients, often without a placebo-control. They are often used to test the safety and effective dose of a substance prior to testing the therapy on a larger group of patients.
Controlled Clinical Trial	This is the most common clinical trial where a selected group is placed upon one of two or more options (placebo, active or test) and followed for an outcome.
Randomized and Blinded	This describes the fact that patients are randomly selected to be placed in each experimental arm and both they and the researcher evaluating their results are blinded to which arm they are in (double-blinded)
Cross-over Design	This describes a study where persons are switched (crossed-over) from one therapy to the other therapy halfway through the trial (from active to placebo or placebo to active). This often allows individuals to act as their own "controls".

Observations and Anecdotes:
Is Seeing Really Believing?

Some of the earliest medical information we have knowledge of is simply the written accounts of observers. The more trained these observers were, the greater and more specific the recorded details. A great many medical discoveries were first recorded by observation, long before our current scientific model confirmed these discoveries with data derived from animal studies and clinical trials. On the other hand, sometimes long-held beliefs and remedies based on recorded observations turn out to be difficult to confirm with modern science, or they are outright debunked. Today, anecdotal evidence and "testimonials" are dismissed as unproven or dubious and held as suspicious by most researchers seeking "evidence-based" outcomes.

As a scientist, I understand and appreciate the need for proper methods of gathering and interpreting data, independent of the bias of the observer(s). Ironically, our new method of data collecting may have its own set of biases and often prevents clinicians from doing what they need to do most—observe patients and listen to their anecdotes. We will explore these assertions further in a moment, but it must be said here that while many modern scientists think they only accept "evidence-based" data, what they often mean is they only accept data that fits the limitations of their understanding and experience, which they believe is free from bias.

Let me give you one example from my own experience. Since the 1980s, glucosamine has been used to treat osteoarthritis and had been studied extensively throughout Europe, Asia, and North America. Through decades of use and dozens of published human clinical trials, few side effects have been observed with glucosamine (rare shellfish allergy potential has been reported) ... but there were *anecdotal* stories that glucosamine might raise blood glucose levels or cause insulin-related issues in diabetic patients. Even though biochemistry tells us that glucosamine cannot be converted to glucose after oral consumption, and several clinical trials specifically designed to ask this question showed no glucose or insulin-related effects whatsoever, even in diabetic patients, several clinicians told me they would still not consider using glucosamine because of the anecdotal "evidence" they had heard.[1] What I find is that anecdotal evidence is accepted or rejected based on whether it agrees with the person's experience. In this case, these clinicians were less familiar with the benefits of glucosamine, so they were very swayed by anything that might be viewed as negative, regardless of the weight of the evidence. Bias, both intentional and unintentional, is a powerful filter affecting how information is transmitted and interpreted. We will give more attention to bias in just a bit.

Population Studies and Epidemiology

As we surveyed in the first two chapters, within the past several centuries we have collected a wealth of health-related population data. This information, coupled with the understanding of disease causation (etiology), has led to the field we call epidemiology. First coined to describe the study of epidemics, epidemiology is the science that attempts to find the relationship between disease patterns, risk factors, and therapeutic interventions. This scientific discipline relies heavily upon previously reported correlations of disease and statistical analysis, with a healthy dose of data adjusting. Of course, this data adjusting is not a "sleight-of-hand" manipulation of the data; it is necessary to make sense of the vast amount of unfiltered data collected. For instance, if we were to compare the death rates of two different populations due to heart disease over a five-year period, one group from France, the other from Australia (each representing 3000 participants), and we simply reported that people from France had twice the number of deaths due to heart disease as people from Australia, this might seem surprising. In our fictional example, this represents the raw, unfiltered, and uninterpreted data. If we reported, however, that the group from Australia was, on average, twenty years younger, 100% women, all treated to guideline-recommended goals for hypertension and lipids, while the French group was 100% male smokers with a previous coronary event, we can see why presenting unadjusted raw data can be problematic.[†]

---

† This result is fictitious. The French Paradox defines France's low risk for heart disease in spite of apparently poor lifestyle decisions. The WHO records an annual heart disease death rate of only 39.8 (per 100,000) in France, compared to 106.9 in the United States and 110.9 in Australia.

While this example is extreme, nearly every health statistic is adjusted or calibrated in some way. Depending on the questions being asked, often dozens of adjustments need to be made to account for age, sex, ethnicity, smoking status, socioeconomic status, education, and the status of numerous laboratory values that increase or decrease the risk for the outcome being measured. Of course, all these adjustments are justified by previous population studies, which themselves have been adjusted for everything but the variable in question (are you following me here?). So if we wanted to know how age affects heart disease, we need to compare a population of individuals and eliminate the influence of everything but age. We must take into account that men and women have different rates of heart disease and adjust for sex, then ethnicity, then smoking status, then LDL-cholesterol level, and so on. In the end, we hope to adjust for everything but age; then we can assume that any difference we see in heart disease rates in different age groups could only be accounted for by age itself. Once the influence of age on heart disease is determined, researchers can use this number to adjust the raw data of other trials and so on (epidemiologists would no doubt cringe at this oversimplification, but it makes the point).

While these adjustments are absolutely critical to make sense of the raw data, researchers can only adjust for variables that are already known to affect the outcome they are measuring. For instance, in a recent weight-loss study it was discovered that two factors were strongly linked to success in losing weight.[2] Those two factors were the sleep duration and the level of perceived stress before and during the weight-loss trial (we will cover the specifics in later chapters). This correlation significantly impacted weight-loss success and was discovered by adjusting the data for everything known to affect weight loss except these two factors. Unfortunately, decades of previous weight-loss clinical trial data cannot be adjusted in the same way to account for these factors unless sleep duration and similar stress measurements were recorded for those patients at the time of those trials. Very often, blood samples are saved for years after the completion of clinical trials so that additional markers, discovered in the future, might be tested in those samples (assuming the biological marker is stable in frozen samples over time). Today, most researchers will publish the unadjusted data, often times with several different levels of adjustment to show how these modifications affect the outcome and conclusions of the clinical trial.

Risk: It's All Relative

From this brief stroll through epidemiology (and trust me, this was a brief stroll), we can see that a vast amount of data, statistical analysis, and biological plausibility is required to make a statement about one activity (smoking, for instance) affecting the risk for a specific disease (cancer). Even with all of this number crunching we still cannot say, with certainty, how this affects the risk in any given individual—only how their risk might compare to the broader population. This is why most population data is described in terms of *relative* risk (RR), or how the risk of certain outcomes for one group is different relative to another group.

Let's see how this works in real life. We will use a study showing the relationship between the consumption of nuts with the risk for diabetes in women. This data was gathered as part of the Nurses' Health Study that included over 83,000 female nurses, followed for 16 years.[3] Starting in 1980, these women filled out information about their current health status, family health history, and diet and physical activity habits. After removing the data from women with previous diabetes or heart disease, they followed this cohort of nurses, asking them to repeat a similar lifestyle and health questionnaire again four times (1984, 1986, 1990, and 1994). Specific to their nut consumption habits, they could choose how often they had consumed a serving of nuts (serving size of 28 g /1 oz.) during the previous year. In the end, they divided this population into four separate groups (quartiles) that they defined based on nut consumption: never, less than 1 oz. per week, 1–4 oz. per week, and greater than 5 oz. per week. Figure 4.1 shows the relative risk for developing diabetes during the sixteen-year follow-up of these women. Because these groups of women are being compared to one another, the researchers set the risk of one group arbitrarily to 1.00; in this case, the group that never consumed nuts has an RR of 1. The risk of each of the other groups of women is then reported *relative* to the first, hence the notion of RR. The numbers reported here show that if we adjust the raw data for the known diabetes risk of age (line 1: age-adjusted RR), the women in the group consuming the most nuts had an RR of 0.55 when compared to the women in the group that never consumed nuts. This RR of 0.55 could also be reported as a 45% lower risk of developing diabetes. When they adjusted these data by the age and body mass index (BMI) of these women—a risk factor strongly associated with developing diabetes—the RR of the highest nut-consumers was now 0.74 (only a 26% reduction in risk; line 2). Then, if the numbers were again adjusted for family history, exercise frequency, smoking status, alcohol consumption, and total calorie intake, something referred to as the "multivariate" relative risk, we had an RR of 0.73 (27% reduction). In this case, the adjustment for age and BMI was so powerful that these other factors added almost nothing to the risk analysis. Now we can conclude, with some degree of confidence, that increased nut consumption for women reduces the risk for diabetes by at least 25%. The authors of the study qualify this by saying, "*Although we cannot rule out the possibility of residual confounding by other potential risk factors, it is unlikely that they can explain the observed inverse association.*" Epidemiologists like to hedge their bets.

Figure 4.1 **Relative Risk from Nurse's Health Study**

	Frequency of Nut Consumption (28-g Serving)				
	Never/ Almost Never	<Once/wk	1–4 Times/wk	≥5 Times/wk	P for Trend
Cases, No.	1314	1133	644	115	...
Person-years	441,007	466,464	309,608	66,468	
Age-adjusted RR (95% CI)	1.00	0.82 (0.76-0.89)	0.69 (0.63-0.76)	0.55 (0.45-0.66)	<.001
Age- and BMI-adjusted RR (95% CI)*	1.00	0.91 (0.84-0.99)	0.83 (0.75-0.91)	0.74 (0.61-0.89)	<.001
Multivariate RR (95% CI)†	1.00	0.92 (0.85-1.00)	0.84 (0.76-0.93)	0.73 (0.60-0.89)	<.001
Additional adjustment for dietary variables, RR (95% CI)‡	1.00	0.91 (0.84-0.99)	0.81 (0.74-0.90)	0.71 (0.57-0.87)	<.001

* BMI indicates body mass index; CI, confidence interval.
† Relative risk was adjusted for age (5-year categories), BMI (<21, 21.0-22.9, 23.0-24.9, 25.0-27.9, 28.0-29.9, 30.0-34.9, ≥35, and missing information), family history of diabetes in a first-degree relative (yes or no), moderate/vigorous exercise (<1, 1, 2-3, 4-6, or ≥7h/wk), cigarette smoking (never, past, or current smoking of 1-14, 15-24, or ≥25 cigarettes/d), alchohol consumption (0, 0.1-5.0, 5.1-15.0, or > 15 g/d), and total energy intake.
‡ Included glycemic load, multivitamin use (yes or no), and intakes of polyunsaturated fat, saturated fat, *trans*-fat, cereal fiber, magnesium, vegetables, fruits, whole grain(in quintiles), and fish (in quartiles).

(Type 2 Diabetes and Nut consumption). See text for explanation.

So understanding how risk is calculated becomes important if we are to recommend starting or stopping certain behaviors to manage risk. If I were asked by a woman concerned about her risk of diabetes, I would tell her that eating nuts (especially almonds, walnuts, and macadamia nuts) is likely to reduce her future risk and, based upon the known evidence, would recommend that she consider doing so. I cannot say from this data alone that diabetes is prevented by eating more nuts; the Nurse's Health study was only observing habits and connecting them with future outcomes. Nut consumption was not used as an intervention in this trial, so we must use other data to make those recommendations.[†]

What's the Significance of All This?

There is nothing more mind-boggling than to hear a room full of epidemiologists and statisticians discuss the meaning of "significance." For research, this is the Holy Grail. Essentially, this term defines whether the data representing two distinct groups is really different or is an artifact of chance. There are many ways to measure statistical significance depending on the type of study being performed. The most commonly used number in medical research is referred to as the "p-value." Essentially the p-value represents the probability that the difference observed between two measurements is real rather than a function of chance. Most commonly, when the p-value is <0.05, we say the data is statistically significant. What this really means is that we are 95% confident that the data does not represent a chance difference.[‡] The smaller the p-value, the higher the confidence we have that chance plays no role in the difference observed between the two outcomes. The p-value for the quartile differences in diabetes risk and nut consumption was <0.001, which represents a 99.9% confidence that this difference is not due to chance. Most would deem these results highly significant.

The statistical significance of a data set is influenced by a number of factors. For clinical research, it is highly influenced by the number of subjects, animals, or units in the groups being studied. This is what we

---

† I can report that numerous intervention trials have been performed with a variety of nut types and doses; most of these trials have shown that nut consumption favorably changes markers of risk for diabetes and related cardio-metabolic disorders. [*Nutrients.* 2010;2(7):652-82.]

‡ Statisticians have a much more nuanced definition of the p-value that includes testing a null hypothesis, but our description has become the *functional* definition for most individuals reading the medical literature.

call the sample size of the experiment (represented by the letter "N"); the larger the number of subjects, the more likely the difference between the subject groups has of reaching statistical significance. The other main factors are related to the magnitude of measurable differences between the groups being compared and how close each individual's measurements compare to the group's average (standard deviation). When the difference is large and the standard deviations are small, the likelihood of statistical significance goes up. It is always important when reading the results of a clinical trial to determine how the measurements of each group are being compared (group average, number of participants reaching a particular goal, etc.) and how the standard deviation for each group affects the confidence that these outcomes are truly different.

Today, scientific research is designed with the end in mind; nothing is left to chance. Statisticians are recruited at the outset of a study to determine how many subjects need to be included to make an expected event reach statistical significance. For instance, if we wanted to study the triglyceride-lowering effects of 1000 mg of omega-3 fatty acids (from fish oil) on individuals with elevated triglycerides (TG), we might start by assuming that a 10% reduction in TG might be achieved in three months with this dose. Based on the confidence interval of similar studies, a statistician can tell us how many subjects would need to finish the three-month trial in order to make our expected 10% difference a statistically significant result. We might find out that the number of subjects is more than the budget will allow (research is expensive). With this information in hand, we could decide to improve our chances for reaching significance by raising the dose (we know that fish oil has a dose-dependent effect on reducing TG), we could choose only the subjects with very elevated TG (the higher the starting number, the greater the TG-lowering effect of most therapies), or we could choose to treat for longer than three months.[4] If our new projected effect is a 20% reduction in TG, we need fewer subjects to reach statistical significance.

Why is this so important? Because all data from clinical trial outcomes is judged solely by the confidence level or statistical significance of the resulting numbers. We will show some interesting examples of how this creates confusion as data is communicated through various channels in a moment.

But Is It Really Significant?

Errors in study design, especially those that do not take into account all the potential factors that can affect statistical significance, create numerous challenges in interpreting the data. When a study shows an important and clinically relevant difference but fails to reach the all-important, pre-determined statistically significant change (perhaps it reaches a p-value of 0.06, just above 0.05), this might be hailed by some as a complete failure and by others as extremely promising data. Depending on who reports the information, the same clinical trial can be presented very differently. If the statistical significance reaches 95% confidence, it might make the evening news, hailed as the next great therapy; if it reaches only 94%, it may be reported as a failed study. Such is the nature of statistics.

In the specter of how scientific studies are presented on the latest morning show or evening news, rarely are these nuances ever mentioned. All we hear is that some activity, food, or drug will double or reduce by half your risk of cancer or some other statement that appears to have an obvious meaning. What if the data supporting the decreased risk associated with consuming a particular food met a high *statistical* significance (say p<0.001) but the difference was of little *clinical* significance? For instance, if the highest consumers of a particular food had three times lower incidence of cancer compared to those who never consumed the food, this would be all over the evening news. If we noted, however, that the incidence of cancer went from three in a million persons to one in a million, we now see that 1/3 of the risk only amounts to two additional persons out of a million individuals. Even if we have enough persons in our sample to make such small differences *statistically* significant, this does not mean the results have a meaningful clinical value. From this data alone, we see that avoiding the food is unlikely to change risk in a real, clinically meaningful way.

When we evaluate studies, we must consider both the statistical and the clinical significance. Is the difference real (not due to chance), and is the difference meaningful (is it clinically relevant)?

The GAIT Keepers: Who Determines if a Trial Succeeds or Fails?

While the adage "Statistics don't lie, but statisticians do" might seem to fit the bill at times, it is often others with an agenda who alter our perception of the data. The following is a story about how study design, statistical significance, and editorial influence can affect how we make clinical decisions. As we noted before, throughout the 1980s and 1990s, the use of glucosamine and/or chondroitin sulfate became very popular for the treatment of osteoarthritis. Research on these compounds was growing, mostly from European research funded by several manufacturers of either glucosamine or chondroitin sulfate. Some of these studies were cell culture studies, which showed how these substances could help chondrocytes (the cells that make cartilage) produce the building blocks of cartilage, and there were also many animal studies. On top of these studies, there were numerous clinical trials in patients with osteoarthritis comparing the effects of glucosamine or chondroitin against placebo and/or pharmaceutical anti-inflammatory agents. While there were many different study designs—some that compared only to placebos, some that compared different doses, some that measured only pain, and some that actually measured changes in joint space—overall they showed a benefit and were, for the most part, statistically significant. But doubt amongst many clinicians in the U.S. still persisted.

Regardless, we were told that these studies had not been performed in the U.S. by "unbiased" researchers, and many clinicians could tell a story (anecdote) of a patient who tried glucosamine or chondroitin and failed to achieve a benefit. So the National Institutes of Health (NIH) decided they would perform a "definitive" trial to answer the question once and for all, to the tune of $12.5 million. The GAIT trial, which stands for **G**lucosamine/**C**hondroitin **A**rthritis **I**ntervention **T**rial, was deemed by the NIH as the "*the first large-scale, multicenter clinical trial in the United States to test the effects of the dietary supplements glucosamine hydrochloride (glucosamine) and sodium chondroitin sulfate (chondroitin sulfate) for the treatment of knee osteoarthritis.*" The goal was to test the ability of glucosamine, chondroitin sulfate, or the combination of the two in reducing pain in patients with knee osteoarthritis after six months of use. They compared these substances to a placebo and a pharmaceutical anti-inflammatory drug (celecoxib/Celebrex) for the same pain outcome.

When the results of the study were announced at the 2005 American College of Rheumatology meeting in San Diego, there was immediate confusion. Some hailed it as a vindication of the benefit of glucosamine and chondroitin, and others claimed the trial proved them to be ineffective. How could this be? To answer this, we need to dig into this just a little bit—but this excursion is well worth the effort if you are serious about understanding how data becomes "evidence" to prove or disprove something.

First of all, the initial report was presented at a scientific meeting in which only some of the data was included. This always allows for selective press reports, quickly written news stories with so-called expert opinions on websites and blogs, long before the nuances of the study are actually published. In this case, the GAIT data was eventually published in the prestigious *New England Journal of Medicine* (*NEJM*) in February of 2006.[5]

A brief discussion of the study design will help here. The researchers in sixteen different clinical centers screened 3238 patients, selecting a total of 1583 subjects with clinically measurable knee osteoarthritis. The average age was 58.6 years, and 64.1% of the subjects were female. These individuals were randomly divided into five groups: P—placebo, G—glucosamine (1500 mg/day), C—chondroitin sulfate (1200 mg/day), G+C—both glucosamine and chondroitin sulfate (at the same doses), and X— celecoxib/Celebrex (200 mg/day). The subjects were followed over 24 weeks for changes in osteoarthritic symptoms, especially joint pain. They were allowed to consume up to 4000 mg of Tylenol (acetaminophen) per day to control pain, if necessary.

Their pre-determined primary outcome (the one that would determine whether the trial "succeeded" or "failed") was a 20% reduction in the WOMAC[†] pain score from baseline to week 24 amongst all

---

† WOMAC stands for Western Ontario and McMaster Universities Osteoarthritis Index and combines 24 different questions pertaining to pain, stiffness, and physical function. A complete description can be found here: http://www.rheumatology.org/practice/clinical/clinicianresearchers/outcomes-instrumentation/WOMAC.asp.

participants. Those who reported this result they called "responders." Researchers predicted (based on previous trials) that the number of responders in the placebo arm would be around 35% and that the dropout rate for each group would be around 20%. With these predictions in hand, they determined that for an intervention to be clinically successful they would need to reach a response rate of 45% (10% greater than the predicted placebo response rate). They selected a statistical threshold of 98.3% (p-value of 0.017 rather than 0.05) to determine significance.

When the trial was completed, researchers reported that the response rate, defined as the percent of individuals achieving a 20% decrease in WOMAC pain score, were as follows (with their respective p-values as each group differed from the placebo group):

> Placebo: 60.1%
> Glucosamine: 64.0% (p=0.30)
> Chondroitin: 65.4% (p=0.17)
> Glucosamine + Chondroitin: 66.6% (p=0.09)
> Celecoxib: 70.1% (p=0.008)

The first thing that should pop out from this data is that while the level of responders in the placebo group was predicted to be 35% before the trial, the actual response for this group was nearly double that level, at 60%. And even though each of the other groups had a greater response rate than researchers originally predicted, only the celecoxib group reached the 10% increase from the placebo and the preset bar of statistical significance. For many, this data was definitive "proof" that neither glucosamine nor chondroitin sulfate was an effective anti-osteoarthritic agent. With that said, the conclusion in the abstract of the *NEJM* article suggested there was more to the story: "*Glucosamine and chondroitin sulfate alone or in combination did not reduce pain effectively in **the overall group of patients** with osteoarthritis of the knee. Exploratory analyses suggest that the combination of glucosamine and chondroitin sulfate may be effective in **the subgroup of patients with moderate-to-severe knee pain**"* [emphasis added]. You might be asking, "What is this exploratory analysis?"

As it turns out, the GAIT investigators rated the osteoarthritis severity for each individual prior to enrolling them in the trial. They divided them into two groups based on pain severity: those with mild pain and those with moderate to severe pain. The secondary analysis (what they call exploratory analysis) showed that in patients with moderate to severe pain, the response rate was much different than the response rate in the overall group of patients (which also included the patients with mild pain), especially between the combination product and celecoxib:

> Placebo: 54.3%
> Glucosamine + Chondroitin: 79.2% (p=0.002)
> Celecoxib: 69.4 % (p=0.06)

In fact, in the moderate to severe pain patients, celecoxib showed no statistical benefit (p=0.06), while the combination of glucosamine and chondroitin showed a highly significant benefit. Unfortunately, the editors and reviewers of the *NEJM* paper limited the conclusion to the primary outcome alone, the results of all the patients combined. Using this information, the combination of glucosamine and chondroitin appears to "fail" and can be reported as a repudiation of these treatments. On the other hand, digging just under the surface of the official conclusions can reveal a result stunningly different than what it might first appear.

Unfortunately most people, including most clinicians, don't have access to the full published articles or the time to read the details of each trial. They, like most Americans, are at the mercy of the authors of the study, the reviewers and editors of the journals, and the media reporting the information: the true "GAIT-keepers."

But the Clinical Trial Said It Would Work!

Perhaps the most profound reality is that no matter how much research we can do, our data can only predict a likely outcome in the average person—and how many "average" people are there? In fact, when we present research data a different way, allowing us to see how each individual in the group responded (rather than just the average of the whole group), we realize that there are many individuals whose results do not reflect the average of the group at all. We call these results or individuals "outliers," because their results lie outside the main group for some reason. So even when the average reduction in LDL-cholesterol amongst hundreds of participants taking a particular agent might be 25%, some individuals within the group might have had a 50% reduction while others a 20% *increase*. The average response of the group does not necessarily predict how each subject will respond.

Researchers know that too many outliers will spoil the experiment. That is, if too many people respond differently than the average and these differences cannot be "adjusted" for, then the chance of reaching statistical significance is compromised. That is why so much effort is taken to have clearly defined inclusion and exclusion criteria. These criteria are used to include individuals who are likely to respond to the therapy or measurement tested while excluding those whose response is less predictable. For instance, if we are testing the effects of a cholesterol-lowering therapy in individuals with elevated LDL-cholesterol, we only want to include those with a predetermined minimum level of LDL-cholesterol; we might want to exclude people who are already on cholesterol-reducing medication, who have a history of poor response to the therapy in question, or who have other known conditions or medications that influence cholesterol metabolism. All of these criteria have been refined from years and years of research, attempting to eliminate the outliers.

In real life, there is no luxury of inclusion and exclusion criteria. Patients enter the clinic with an assortment of conditions, previous therapies, and current medications. This is even more so when dealing with a chronic health condition. Their outcome is neither "the average" nor "the outlier," since this is an experiment where N=1. On top of that, almost never is the clinical setting as controlled as a clinical trial, in which everything is measured and adjusted for in order to optimize statistical outcomes. Simply put, a patient is not a controlled clinical trial.

I am reminded of this fact all the time when discussing specific patient outcomes with clinicians. One particular example would be the many questions concerning the effectiveness of certain nutrients or drugs for the support of bone mineral density (BMD) in post-menopausal women. The conversation starts something like this: "I have a patient—a 51-year-old woman—a year into menopause, I have had her using your product for a year, and her BMD is 3% lower than it was a year ago. The studies say these ingredients should increase her BMD by

2%. I think the product is defective, and my patient is upset." What follows is a bit of the explanation I use with this common complaint:

The loss of bone density and strength and fracture risk has been fairly well documented in postmenopausal women for years. The figure below shows the average bone mass in both men and women based on age.

Figure 4.2. **Bone Mass over time in men and women**

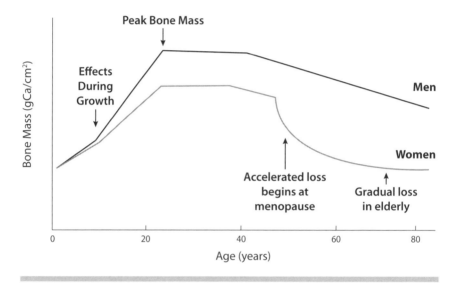

As you can easily see, the rate of bone mass reduction immediately following menopause in women is dramatically steep. With no specific intervention, this rate of bone loss continues for several years and tapers off to a steady but less dramatic decline after a decade or so. Researchers attempting to test the effects of nutrients or drugs on changes in BMD in postmenopausal women have known for years that they must control for these differences. Very often, women are excluded from trials unless they have passed the menopausal transition for enough years to reach the "slower" decline (typically three to five years or more). This inclusion/exclusion is fairly typical of clinical trials for osteoporosis-related nutrients and drugs, although these details are usually glossed over by almost everyone reporting the information.

Few clinical trials would choose women just entering menopause to test a therapy for improving BMD because bone turnover is so unstable and affected by many factors that are difficult to adjust for. After this discussion and with this additional information in mind, the clinician realizes that a 3% decrease in BMD during the initial phase of post-menopausal bone loss may actually represent a *better* course of events than what may have occurred had the patient not taken the product at all. Of course we don't have the luxury of going backwards a year and seeing what the natural course of bone density changes would have been, a sort of placebo-controlled trial to compare the current results. When we add to the discussion other factors that influence BMD like stress-induced cortisol production, gastrointestinal absorption of nu-trients, weight, physical activity, diet, pharmaceuticals, and more, the practice of chronic disease management emerges as the complex matrix that it really is. Once again, we realize that a person is never just "the average" participant in a controlled clinical trial, and we mustn't treat them as if they are.

While most clinics don't simply turn away patients who are likely to be outliers, over time clinics begin to specialize in certain patient types that are often a self-selected group seeking out their help. Eventually, this may alter the "inclusion criteria" of those on the waiting list. I of-ten hear clinicians say things like, "My patients are all post-menopausal women looking for alternatives to conventional hormone replacement therapy." Sometimes clinicians have inclusion and exclusion criteria, perhaps under a different name, to control the outliers amongst their patient populations.[†]

Evaluating Scientific Studies: The Bottom Line

I think you can now see just a bit of the reason scientific research can confuse even the most studious of persons. The more we know, the

---

† Perhaps you are reading this and feeling that you might be an outlier, the patient who is being shifted from practice to practice. You have undergone every test that has been invented, twice, with no answer, and your full-time job has become your own health situa-tion. You've read every book that might hold the secret answer to your condition—and still no solution. Things seem to work for a time, but then they fail, and the situation feels worse than before. Don't give up hope—the answer likely lies in a synergistic approach that can't be achieved by a single "magic bullet" solution.

more it seems we still don't know. Scientific meetings are routinely filled with panel discussions and outright debates, where various camps interpret the same data with vastly different, even opposing, conclusions. Let me give just a few parting suggestions as you attempt to wade further into research studies and the recommendations derived from their conclusions.

- Always ask the basic questions when you hear about a new clinical trial.
  - What type of study was this?
  - What types of patients were included, and which ones were excluded?
  - What was the outcome, and how long did it take?
  - Was the result clinically significant?
  - What were the side effects?
  - What are the criticisms of the study, and are they legitimate?
  - How does this study compare to others of similar design?
  - Is there a plausible biological explanation for the results?

- Guideline recommendations are always an outcome derived by the consensus of many individuals and studies, often after years of compromise. One or two influential individuals can impact the recommendations of a whole panel of participants. Always check the date of the guideline recommendations you are using; often they are ten or more years old, using only the data that garnered a consensus at the time.

- Don't forget about what already works. In our rush to keep up with the latest research, we often forget about all the therapies that are tried and true. This is characteristic of both clinician and patient; we all love the shiny new toy. The best therapy is often not the newest.

- Remember the outlier. No matter how clinically and statistically significant the outcome, some individuals simply will not respond or will respond in the opposite fashion from the average (approved sleeping pills give some people insomnia!).

- Media reports will always hype a story beyond the implications of the actual study results. Few things are as great or horrible as they are first reported.

- There is no such thing as unbiased research. This doesn't mean that there isn't honest and good research amongst those with a bias; it just means that we need to be aware of the conflicts of interest that exist amongst those who fund, perform, interpret, publish, and promote a study. Even as readers, we might have a bias by selecting which studies we read in detail and which we ignore.

Even if you don't understand every new scientific discovery, you can still sift through the latest health report or late-night infomercial with a critical eye. In the end, the more you know about how scientific information is gathered, adjusted, and disseminated, the better you'll be able to put it in context and decide how to leverage it for your benefit.

CHAPTER 5

Vis medicatrix naturae
The Healing Power
of the Body

"It is highly dishonorable for a reasonable soul to live in so divinely built a mansion as the body she resides in—altogether unacquainted with the exquisite structure of it."
—Robert Boyle (1627–1691)

OUR HEALTH IS A complex relationship between our genetics and our decisions, nature and nurture working together. It can be influenced by what our mother ate while we were in utero or by what we ate last night. Rarely is it determined by a single gene or a single event but instead by the cumulative effects of thousands upon thousands of decisions we make every day and how our genes and cells respond to those decisions. Knowing how our body interprets those decisions and choices and turns them into signals of health or disease will help us leverage the power of our own choices. In other words, our health is not determined by the cards we're dealt but by the way we play the hand.

Now that you are armed with the basic historical and scientific landscape of lifestyle medicine, we want to turn the corner and delve deeper into the subject. We have already seen what the combination of poor lifestyle choices can do to the health of a person and a population;

now we need to take a few steps and ask ourselves, why? What causes good or bad lifestyle decisions to affect health or disease? What are the driving mechanisms causing the rapid increase of metabolic diseases like obesity and diabetes? And just how does our body take in the information it receives from food, sleep, physical activity, and stress and turn this into changes that we later call disease or health? If we understood the answers to these questions, or even knew how to find the answers, we would have the key to the mystery and power of lifestyle as medicine. And with that, we can unlock the gate leading to the prevention and reversal of most chronic diseases plaguing our nation.

In order to begin this process, we need to jump a little deeper into the basic physiological and genetic processes that make us function; to do that, we must first separate and lay out some key concepts before building the whole model. Each of these concepts is a subject of numerous papers and books, with details and nuances that can be quite complex. However, we will keep our discussion limited to those portions that are needed to build our model and leave some of the nuances for you to explore on your own, if you choose. For those with a bit less background in scientific research, especially biology, some of these concepts might seem difficult to follow at first, but once we begin using them to explain how they impact health, these principles will become quite a bit clearer. Ironically, many of today's clinicians went through medical school before some of these ideas were even explored and are themselves learning some of these concepts for the first time in recent days.

Vis medicatrix naturae

Let's start off with a very old and basic observation: the human body has an amazing ability to heal itself. You don't need to know much about the intricacies of the immune system or molecular biology to appreciate this reality. This notion of self-healing is rooted in a much larger phenomenon: that of self-preservation. To put it simply, "life" is imprinted at every level of our being, while death is an intruder. Life, by its very essence, is self-sustaining. From the Judeo-Christian perspective, with which I am most familiar, "life" speaks of more than merely a physical existence but something much deeper—something superimposed upon our biology.† The "will to live," as we might call it, often seems to trump physiology. But how does this concept of "life" translate into physiological events that actually preserve us and keep us healthy?

The Latin phrase *vis medicatrix naturae* is often used by natural healing traditions to teach this phenomenon: that the "healing mechanism" is an intrinsic property of our body.[1] What this "healing mechanism" is and how it works are obviously explained in different ways by these many traditions, most of them having done so well before the benefit of modern scientific research. Now, after the benefit of decades of scientific research, from epidemiology to epigenetics, we can still say, without a doubt, that the intrinsic healing potential resident within our body is far and away the most powerful medical tool we possess. It is a tool we too often let languish as we look past what the body can do by itself and toward what are perceived as more powerful drugs and surgical procedures to "fix the cause of the disease."

It has been said that "*the art of medicine consists of amusing the patient while nature cures the disease*".‡ And while we don't mean to trivialize the vast knowledge and skill set of today's clinician, sometimes the job of a masterful clinician is to provide only the necessary elements that allow the patient's body to heal itself. So powerful is this healing mechanism that clinical trials are not considered valid unless they are "controlled" by giving a placebo to one group (unbeknownst to them) in order to subtract this influence, which is often so strong it prevents the tested therapy from reaching statistical significance. Among other things, the placebo response has taught us that many of the improvements seen after clinical intervention can be attributed wholly or partially to this intrinsic healing property of the body. Even many clinical

---

† From a Judeo-Christian perspective, this is realized when the human spirit is incorporated into the human body, generating a unique form of life neither portion can attain without the other. The account of Adam's creation includes both the formation of his body (from the ground) and the breath of God (spirit), which caused him to become a living being (soul).

‡ This particular translation of the quote is attributed to the French philosopher Voltaire (1694–1778), although similar phrases have been attributed to others perhaps stemming from the statement from Hippocrates (460 BC–377 BC): "*Everyone has a physician inside him or her; we just have to help it in its work. The natural healing force within each one of us is the greatest force in getting well.*"

guidelines often describe a "watch and wait" approach, acknowledging that many conditions are "self-limiting." These, of course, are modern scientific ways to say that we have no intervention with a better risk-reward outcome than what the body can do on its own.

If we combine the power of *vis medicatrix naturae,* our body's own healing potential, with understanding from the latest research defining the mechanisms of chronic disease, we can absolutely revolutionize the current paradigm of medicine and unleash the power of lifestyle medicine as it was intended. This approach opens a whole new set of questions that Koch's postulates could never address: What mechanisms allow our body to convert the thousands upon thousands of input signals into healthy (or unhealthy) outcomes? What are the most powerful health-promoting signals? Does everyone have the same natural healing capacity? Will the same inputs be good for everyone? How much abuse can the system tolerate before it stops working? And can you improve your natural healing capacity? Let's explore this further.

Our bodies are designed to take the appropriate messages from our "lifestyle" and turn them into "health." Since the most powerful remedy is the intrinsic healing mechanism within our bodies, therapies will work best when they are targeted toward triggering these mechanisms rather than circumventing them.

Fundamental to the process of sustaining life in the face of a potential mortal threat is prioritizing those functions that are vital for immediate survival over those that are not. Under stressful situations, say something like running from an attacking grizzly bear, maintaining optimal long-term bone mineral density is of little immediate concern. Proper bone turnover performed by osteoblast and osteoclast metabolism is unlikely to save your life in this particular case.[†] Fast-forward a few decades and the repeated neglect of bone mineralization can make you vulnerable to a life-threatening fracture.[2] This illustration teaches us an important lesson: our bodies use a sort of "triage" method to decide

---

[†] This is for illustrative purposes only; this book is not a "survival guide." Running from a grizzly is only recommended when you are with a companion who is sufficiently slower than you. Please see more about the consequences of the stress response in chapter 10.

which functions are of immediate life-saving importance, suspending other important functions which are not needed to solve the immediate crisis.† If those important long-term functions remain neglected for too long or undergo frequent suspension, chronic dysfunction will be followed by chronic disease. As we will see while building the Lifestyle Synergy Model, our long-term health is a delicate balance between solving immediate needs and at the same time maintaining enough resources for a healthy future.

The Homeostatic Model

One of the classic concepts used to describe the body's own healing capacity is homeostasis. This is the idea that the body has a "steady-state," or set point, and a series of mechanisms to maintain this set point. Homeostasis is sometimes viewed like a thermostat that turns on either the heating or the cooling system to maintain a fixed temperature. We are told, for instance, that "normal" body temperature is 37° Celsius (98.6° Fahrenheit), and deviations from normal often signal a problem. Actually, "normal" body temperature is not a fixed number but follows a subtle curve throughout the day and even throughout the month (especially in premenopausal women). In fact, body temperature is rarely ever "normal," being constantly adjusted by time of day, hormone levels, metabolic needs, room temperature, and physical activity. The complexities of the processes that maintain body temperature (thermoregulation) are just one part of the many inter-related, fluctuating systems within our bodies. Ironically, there are actually very few truly "steady-states" in biological systems.

The Greek term "homeostasis" was first applied to these biological functions in the days when we had only crude measuring tools unable to detect subtle changes in many bodily functions. As with body temperature, however, subtle fluctuation and sometimes wide-ranging oscillating patterns are actually the norm for most biological systems. Frequently these fluctuations track along a circadian rhythm, while others

---

† We use the notion of physiological triage here in a similar, but slightly different, way as Bruce Ames, who describes his triage theory of allocating scarce resources (vitamins/antioxidants) in order to preserve the life of the organism [*PNAS* November 21, 2006;103(47):17589-17594].

follow specific events (such as eating or stress); for some the controlling mechanisms are still unknown. For instance, in a normal, healthy person the stress hormone cortisol might be ten times higher when they awaken than it is while they sleep at 2 AM.[3] We rarely think of this sort of variation when we think of homeostasis, but, in fact, this is normal. Perhaps another term should be used to describe this phenomenon, one that encompasses its rhythmic, dynamic, and reactive characteristics.

One interesting example of this phenomenon is heart rate variability (HRV), which describes the variability in the time intervals between each heartbeat at rest. It was not until the 1960s that we had the ability to even detect the subtle fluctuations in timing of the beating heart, discovering a link with heart disease risk. In fact, the less variability between each heartbeat, the higher the risk for death, hypertension, heart disease, diabetes, and a number of related disease outcomes.[4] So here is a clear case where a rhythmic variability, undetectable before the tools of modern technology, actually helps define healthy function (in this case, a healthy balance between the sympathetic and parasympathetic nervous systems).[5] We should mention before leaving this example that HRV is adversely affected by a number of lifestyle factors, such as obesity, physical inactivity, and smoking, also known to drive chronic disease.[6]

We need to recognize that the key to maintaining our health lies with our body's capacity to maintain the rhythmic and reactive nature of these dynamic homeostatic mechanisms. And maintaining the integrity of these mechanisms is dependent upon receiving and interpreting a host of physiological signals. Some of those signals come from within our bodies, while the rest come from the outside world. The majority of the signals that train and maintain these mechanisms, not surprisingly, are those we provide through diet, physical activity, sunlight, sleep, and a host of other lifestyle-related activities. The good or bad signals that we provide help or hurt our ability to stay healthy and therefore increase or inhibit the benefit we get when using other interventions like supplements, chiropractic care, and physical therapy—even drugs and surgery.

Lifestyle medicine is not about doing the same exact thing every day but about understanding the rhythms and responses that our body uses to keep us healthy. When our actions mirror this understanding, we create a synergistic force that unlocks the healing power within each cell. We must work with our body, not impose a solution upon it.

Physiological Resiliency: To Bend without Breaking

So, if the ability to maintain health is a design feature built into our bodies, why don't we just remain healthy all the time? This might seem obvious when we think of major external threats such as trauma (car accidents, gunshot wounds), invading organisms (viruses, bacteria), or major genetic defects that result in a compromised metabolic machinery. But aside from these major types of events, what accounts for the drift from health to disease that seems to be inseparable from normal aging and is creeping into the experience of younger and younger individuals as each decade passes? To answer this, we need to discuss an important concept that I call physiological resiliency, or the "buffers" that each cell and organ system rely upon to compensate when things go wrong. And things will definitely go wrong.

Physiological resiliency is built into nearly every level of complexity in our bodies, from the enzymes designed to scan DNA for damage before a cell divides to the process that allows sleep to reset the stress-response system. Simply put, our bodies have an amazing capacity to buffer unfavorable events and recover when things go awry. These overlapping systems, each with their own regulatory mechanisms, are constantly adjusting and readjusting based on thousands of input signals that come from inside and outside our bodies. Like a rubber band or coiled spring, these mechanisms have a given resiliency that creates a "bend but don't break" system. But just like a rubber band, overstretching the system time and time again is not without its consequences.

To unpack this concept further, let's start with the basics of how a buffering system works. We often think of buffering systems in chemistry when we are attempting to maintain a steady concentration of a particular ion. One of the most important chemical buffering systems in the body helps control the pH of our blood. Keeping the appropriate acid-base balance in the blood is crucial for immediate survival—we simply cannot function very well when our blood strays away from the optimal pH of 7.4. This highly regulated pH is needed to maintain the appropriate environment for enzymatic reactions in the bloodstream and tissues.

Since the blood pH is so critical, this buffering system has a very narrow range and must be tightly monitored to keep us alive. In this case, we have a carbonic acid-bicarbonate buffering system that involves both kidney and lung function. When we are physically active and our muscles require more oxygen and energy, they produce H+ (hydrogen ions) and CO_2 (carbon dioxide); when these compounds diffuse into the circulation, the carbonic acid/bicarbonate buffering capacity of the blood compensates for these changes while the lungs and kidneys help to reset the buffering capacity of the blood. Many events can trigger the need for the blood pH buffering system, including the basic metabolic functions of all cells, changes in temperature, some foods,[†] some supplements, stress, infections, and certain pharmaceutical agents. It is critical that these factors do not alter the blood pH, hence the need for the buffering system. If the buffering system is unprepared for sharp alterations in blood pH, a major health emergency quickly ensues—there is little room for error. On the other hand, some tissues in the body function better at pH ranges that differ from the blood—some slightly more alkaline, some slightly more acidic, and some greatly more acidic (like the stomach at a pH of 2). Each cell maintains its own buffering capacity that is, in turn, enhanced by the blood's buffering system.

Blood pH is a true acid-base buffering system, but a number of other biological systems fulfill the general definition of a buffer we are trying to explain. Another important system we could describe as an overlapping buffering system is the highly coordinated antioxidant system our bodies use to prevent oxidative damage to our tissues. Normal cellular activities produce billions of highly reactive intermediate chemical spe-

---

† There is quite a large discussion about foods that "acidify" and others that "alkalize" the blood. Most of these foods or dietary patterns have not been rigorously tested, but it does appear from some small studies that ingested foods and beverages can deplete or increase the blood's buffering capacity, pushing blood pH towards an acidic or alkaline level.

cies called free radicals. These free radical compounds are important and necessary for the functioning of the cell, but they are highly reactive and must be tightly controlled to preserve the integrity of the cell.

A complex network of antioxidants is designed to prevent these reactive intermediates from damaging cells and tissues. Some of these antioxidants are enzymes (superoxide dismutase), some antioxidants are produced in the cell by enzymes (glutathione), some we must ingest (vitamins E and C), and some actually induce the production of the enzymes that then produce antioxidants (sulforophane from broccoli). In a few cases, like the powerful antioxidant compound lipoic acid, agents can act directly as antioxidants, indirectly by re-charging other antioxidants (in this case vitamin E, vitamin C, and glutathione), and by inducing antioxidant enzyme systems.[7] Lipoic acid has become a very important and popular nutraceutical supplement for this reason.

Since the burden of unquenched free radicals forms the basis for one of the leading theories of the cause of aging and chronic disease progression, the strength of our antioxidant network is critical to our overall health and our aging process. Decisions we make about our diet, physical activities, and environmental exposure can play a tremendous role in depleting or expanding the antioxidant buffering capacity we enjoy and, in turn, the physiological resilience of the systems that maintain our health.

Now I would like to extend the term "buffer" to more complex systems so we can get a better understanding of the mechanisms that produce the physiological resilience we rely upon. Unlike blood pH, which is maintained within a fairly tight window (closer to the original definition of homeostasis), blood *glucose* levels must necessarily rise and fall in response to food consumption and metabolic needs. In fact, the rise in blood glucose triggers an increase in the production of insulin that is critical for glucose transport into many cells. So in this case, we need to have a responsive system that allows for a transient increase in blood glucose with a compensatory rise in insulin to drive this important energy source throughout the body and into cells needing glucose.

Maintaining appropriate blood glucose levels throughout the day is a highly coordinated effort involving numerous organ systems, hormones, cell signaling mechanisms, and intracellular metabolic processes.

Figure 5.1 below shows three basic patterns of blood glucose changes throughout the day. Note the rise in blood glucose after each meal (post-prandial), followed by a gradual decline to baseline. This rise and fall is called the glucose excursion after a meal. This glucose excursion is dependent upon a number of factors: the total amount of food we consume, the glycemic impact of that food, and the physiologic resilience of our blood glucose regulating processes. If we have normal physiological resilience and insulin sensitivity, when we consume a meal our blood glucose (and insulin) rises and falls in a predictable timeframe. Years and years of eating meals that strain the glycemic response (with meals containing high amounts of calories from refined carbohydrates and

Figure 5.1 Blood Glucose Excursions Based on Glucose Tolerance

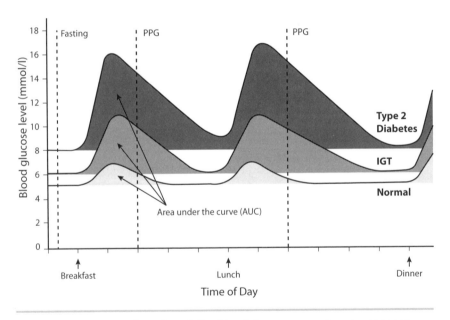

These three curves show the relative blood glucose excursions in response to typical meals throughout the day for individuals with normal glucose tolerance, impaired glucose tolerance, or diagnosed type 2 diabetes. Fasting glucose is usually measured after an overnight fast, while post-prandial glucose (PPG) is typically measured 2 hours after consuming a meal. Note the large difference in the area under the curve (AUC) for glucose in these types of individuals, relative to the much smaller differences in fasting glucose levels.

saturated fats and absent of fiber, micronutrients, and insulin-sensitizing phytonutrients) and we drift away from this tight control.

As we stretch the buffering systems and move from normal glucose tolerance to "impaired" glucose tolerance (IGT), notice in the figure that there is only a small change in the baseline, or fasting, blood glucose levels. If we were to only measure fasting glucose levels, a classic measure of homeostasis, we would be fooled into thinking little was happening, when in fact the size of the glucose excursion (measured by the area under the curve, AUC) has greatly increased. As this continues for decades, the physiological resilience, like a rubber band, continues to be stretched until it is unable to bring even the fasting glucose into safe ranges, resulting in a diagnosis of type 2 diabetes, along with a host of rogue glucose-related reactions that damage sensitive tissues.

One of the hallmarks of metabolic aging is a drift—or to use our analogy, a stretching of the rubber bands—that keeps a tight rein on the daily glucose excursions. Along with many other changes that occur during aging, it is not merely the direction of the change but rather the speed at which the change occurs that overwhelms us. Again—this system is built with a buffer—our cells can tolerate a reasonable number of changes and adapt to them quite nicely. With few exceptions, we are born with enough buffering capacity to withstand the subtle metabolic drifts that come with aging if we choose enough of the right signals to keep our resilience strong. Researchers continue to tell us that these pathophysiological changes are well characterized and nearly 100% preventable if we make the right choices in life. The daily drivers of metabolic resilience are tied to the amounts and types of foods we consume, the types and frequency of the physical activities we engage in, the level of stress we experience, the amount of sleep we get, and a host of other lifestyle and environmental factors that we choose on a daily basis. Our ability to improve the mechanisms driving glucose intolerance and metabolic drift is in our own hands (or mouths).

Fat Mass: The Ultimate Buffer Gone Awry

As we mentioned briefly in chapter 2, the current obesity epidemic represents the cumulative stretching of the buffering capacity of the entire body. In a very fundamental way, adipose tissue (fat) is specifically designed to help buffer the ebb and flow of nutrient availability. When feast is followed by famine, this buffer is a means of survival; when feast is followed by more feasting, however, then our buffer system may not know how to turn itself off. So when blood sugar rises, our adipose tissue is capable of removing the immediate danger to sensitive tissues by converting glucose into fat and storing it for the future. When stress induces high levels of the hormone cortisol, adipose tissue is also activated to store more fat. When fat-soluble toxins accumulate in the body, they build up in adipose tissue; some toxins even stimulate fat production. In fact, adipose tissue can be stimulated by any number of signals to increase the storage of fat. It is in many ways the body's ultimate buffering system.

As such, its capacity for fat storage in humans seems to be without limit but not without consequence. Since the body is designed to treat the stored fat as a buffer for future needs, it has mechanisms to protect the accumulated adipose tissue. In fact, when someone loses fat mass while dieting, they actually trigger the brain to think they are in crisis, often promoting an increased desire to eat and a metabolic shift toward heightened fat production. This is a normal part of how the body attempts to preserve its buffering system. If you have ever lost a lot of weight, you know how hard your body tries to hold onto fat. Our buffers have a limit: if we bend them too far, they will break.

Our bodies are designed with a series of overlapping buffering mechanisms that give us an amazing resilience against poor lifestyle decisions. Every lifestyle decision we make strengthens or weakens the capacity of this system a little bit at a time. It may take months, years, or even decades to notice, but both good and bad decisions have a cumulative effect on our ability to create a healthy outcome.

Is There a Point of No Return?

The physiological resilience we have outlined here could be described for hundreds of different biological processes in our bodies. We have discussed briefly the ones involving blood pH, blood sugar, adipose accumulation, thermo-regulation, and the antioxidant system; but nearly every important biological function has a complex buffer-type system intended to keep the organism within a window of viability and function. Some of these systems are tightly controlled; others have quite a bit more flexibility. Unfortunately, each of these buffering systems has a limit.

We will illustrate this point by using our previous example of blood glucose. As we discussed, the ability to return blood sugar to normal fasting levels (~70–80 mg/dl) after eating a meal is generally referred to as glucose tolerance. In fact, there is a standard way to measure someone's glucose tolerance using what is called an oral glucose tolerance test (OGTT), which measures a person's blood sugar and insulin for several hours after consuming a specific amount of glucose. There are a number of factors that determine a person's glucose tolerance, but we will focus on just two for the sake of simplicity: the person's overall sensitivity to insulin (or conversely their insulin resistance) and the actual amount of insulin produced by the pancreas in response to consuming glucose.

Notice in Figure 5.2 what is often referred to as "the metabolic continuum." As time passes, most of us move along this continuum toward progressively higher insulin resistance, some more quickly than others. Essentially, this tells us that the mechanisms that cause insulin to trigger glucose transport into cells are becoming less responsive to insulin. Insulin resistance results in higher post-prandial blood glucose, and

Figure 5.2 **The Metabolic Continuum**

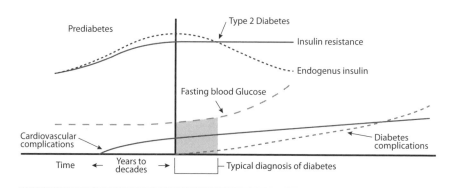

This figure shows the general progression over time of insulin resistance and insulin production. Notice that fasting blood glucose only becomes high enough to be considered "diabetes" once the endogenous insulin production ceases to increase in compensation with the continued insulin resistance.

because the cells are less responsive to insulin, your body also requires higher production of insulin to bring the blood glucose down to baseline levels. The continual stretching of this system slowly pushes the baseline fasting blood glucose higher and higher. It may take decades of poor eating habits to push normal fasting blood glucose levels from 80 mg/dl to pre-diabetic levels of over 100 mg/dl in the average person. All the while, the beta cells in the pancreas are working harder and harder to produce more insulin because the peripheral cells (especially adipose tissue and muscle tissue) are becoming less responsive to the insulin being produced. This is the drift of the metabolic continuum.

Now what happens when the pancreatic beta cells themselves begin to succumb to the growing demands caused by their need to produce so much insulin? Actually, we know what happens, and it is not good. Initially these cells begin to grow in size (hypertrophy) in response to the demand to produce more insulin. They adjust, as we would expect, to this increased demand as they were designed to do. However, these changes put a higher oxidative burden on the cell, slowly depleting the cell's antioxidant buffering capacity. Not only does this process contribute to the dysfunction of beta cells, it actually begins leading to the very destruction of these cells by way of programmed cell death, a process called apoptosis.[8] When all the buffering capacities of the cell are exhausted, the cell just dies.

When we combine this depleting insulin production of the pancreas with the continued insulin resistance of the peripheral tissue, the math just doesn't add up, and there is simply no place for the blood sugar to go. So what was at first a gradual increase in fasting blood glucose, perhaps not even worth mentioning after looking at a routine lab test, all of a sudden becomes a crisis and a diagnosis of type 2 diabetes. Once this critical inflection point is crossed, the process becomes much more difficult to correct, but it is still a long way from being irreversible. We do know, however, that the longer someone has been diagnosed with type 2 diabetes, even while being treated with pharmaceutical anti-diabetic drugs, the more their pancreatic beta cell function continues to deteriorate until they reach a point where insulin therapy itself is required to bring blood glucose levels outside of dangerous levels. Usually by that time hyperglycemia has done most of its damage to the cardiovascular system and is well on its way to damaging a host of microvascular tissues in the eyes, kidneys, and nervous system.

Perhaps a word picture can best illustrate how we can understand the continuum that leads us further and further toward irreversibility. Imagine you are rowing a canoe across a wide body of water. So wide is this body of water that you assume it to be a quiet lake. Actually, you are not in a lake but instead in a wide area of a deep, flowing river. Since the current is not strong, you can easily paddle downstream or upstream with little effort; but if you stopped paddling for a while, you would notice that you drifted ever so slowly downstream—this is the beginning of the metabolic continuum. The current is gentle, in fact hardly noticeable; it only really carries you along if you stop paddling altogether. Now assume that we let the current slowly move us downstream into a narrower part of the river where the current is a bit stronger. Paddling against the current now becomes a chore, but moving further downstream takes very little effort. "No problem," you say. After all, the river is beautiful and the canoe seems fine; so far, so good. At this point going with the flow seems to be a lot less work than paddling upstream—you're busy with life anyway—so the canoe, or the metabolic continuum, speeds up.

If our illustration had a soundtrack, at this point you would begin hearing the distant roar of rushing water. Out of sight and around the bend in our metabolic "river of life" is a drop-off with a few well-placed rocks. Concerned about your ability to navigate these rapids, you begin paddling fervently upstream. It is only then that you realize the current is much faster and stronger than you had imagined; when did that happen? With a concerted effort you might be able to maintain your position; with a heroic effort you might even be up to paddling upstream and out of the way of danger. It's pretty obvious where this illustration is going.

After your arms wear out from paddling, your canoe succumbs to the current, and now you turn your attention away from paddling upstream to navigating through the rapids without damaging or tipping your canoe over. It's a difficult stretch, you take in some water, but you make it to the bottom relatively unscathed. After relaxing for a few moments you realize that some of your provisions must have fallen out of the canoe as you navigated the rapids in haste, and others are water-logged. Your provisions for the future (your buffers) are now

damaged or lost. After a while, however, you forget about these triviali-
ties—thankful once again that the river appears to be quiet. Between
each set of rapids a new "set-point" is reached and a new "normal" becomes the reality. Getting back upstream is not impossible, but without
a concerted effort and plan it is unlikely. Metabolic drift is much like
this river: if we maintain our position when we are strong and full of
provisions, we won't have to paddle upstream to avoid danger. Our illustration could go on and on, repeating this scenario numerous times
until finally the river plunges down a rocky ravine, forming a deadly
waterfall—the final and truly irreversible event in our canoe trip.

Years ago, I developed a product to help support individuals suffering from chronic venous insufficiency and varicose veins. It was a blend
of herbs known to be helpful in preventing some of the mechanisms
and symptoms related to these conditions.[†] I was always asked, "Can
this product reverse varicose veins?" What usually ensued was a long
discussion of how vessel tone is controlled and how varicose veins form.
This included the explanation of the four different layers that make up
the vessel wall, including the specialized cells that create valves along the
lumen of the vessel to help move blood in one direction from your feet to
your heart, defying gravity. I often explained that once a particular valve
is compromised and unable to prevent blood from flowing back down
to the next valve, it is virtually irreversible; however, it is eminently possible to reverse the *process* that leads to further varicosities by improving
vessel tone. As with most chronic health concerns, once you're below the
rapids, paddling upstream becomes much harder—sometime impossible. The power of the Lifestyle Synergy Model is to help you reverse the
process that drives chronic disease, slowing the river and strengthening
your ability to paddle upstream at the same time.

Metabolic Reserve: Our Long-Term Buffering Capacity

Now we want to explore a very specific and important aspect of
physiological resilience, something we will refer to as metabolic reserve.

---

† This product contained extracts of horsechestnut (seed), butcher's broom (root), and gotu kola
(leaf) with something called troxerutin, a flavonoid extract. It was the first such combination of
these powerful agents in the U.S., and the formula remains basically the same to this day.

Essentially, this defines the combined reserve capacity of the various buffering systems used to maintain key critical functions or organ systems in the body. A subset of the idea of metabolic reserve is sometimes called organ reserve, which defines the buffering capacity of a particular organ or organ system to maintain itself. It should be noted that in most cases there is no specific measuring tool that can gauge the strength of each particular organ system's reserve, so this concept is not widely discussed in the current healthcare model.[†]

Let us give a fairly straightforward example of this idea using bone mineral density (BMD). Normally, we become concerned about BMD in the context of post-menopausal women and osteoporosis. But as Figure 5.3 shows, BMD follows a somewhat predictable pattern over a woman's lifetime. The shape of this curve is somewhat similar for every woman, but the exact measurements of the peaks and valleys are not predetermined by genetics or age alone.

Figure 5.3 **Bone Mass in Women and Men Over Time**

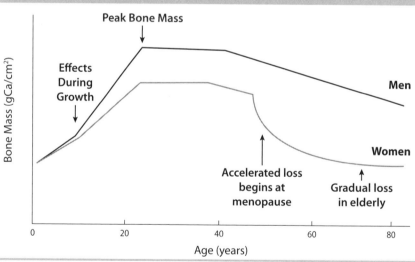

The general shape of this curve is similar in all women, but the height of peak bone mass and the slope of the bone loss later in life is determined by thousands of lifestyle decisions over her life.

† The notion of metabolic reserve has been used elsewhere in a similar fashion. Two prominent ways metabolic reserve is defined are 1) the athletic capacity (or reserve) that elite athletes have available in critical performance situations and 2) the heart's capacity (reserve) to respond to increases in workload demand.

Most people focus their attention on the rapid acceleration in bone loss that begins at menopause. There are numerous drugs and hundreds of clinical trials attempting to slow this decline or rebuild the BMD once it settles to its new set point after menopause. While it's certainly important to slow or even reverse the loss of BMD in post-menopausal women (something that is possible without pharmaceutical intervention), one of the most important keys to preventing osteoporosis is something that precedes this by more than thirty years. Long before most women are even thinking about osteoporosis, they are establishing their greatest potential protection against it by building their peak bone mass.[9] As the quintessential picture of a metabolic or organ reserve, peak bone mass serves as a special sort of buffer against the eventual decline that occurs decades later.

Not surprisingly, building peak BMD is dramatically influenced by years of lifestyle decisions, mostly when a woman is between her early teens and early thirties. Diet is key, of course, but so is the amount and type of physical activity she participates in, her amount of sunlight exposure (or vitamin D consumed), abstinence from unhealthy habits such as smoking, and even the amount of stress she is burdened with (remember our story about the grizzly bear and building bone mass). Like paddling upstream in the wide part of the river, building metabolic reserve takes full advantage of, and even strengthens, our physiological reserve and our healing capacity. On the other hand, while clinically appropriate in many situations, pharmaceutical drugs rarely if ever build metabolic reserve, and often their side effects are a direct result of depleting metabolic reserve.†

Our example of BMD is quite straightforward and easy to measure, but this principle can be applied to nearly every system of the body. Think about the metabolic reserve of the liver in its capacity to detoxify, or the brain's ability to maintain its efficiency to store and recall memo-

---

† Some of the most popular drugs used to "treat" osteoporosis actually inhibit the process of normal bone turnover and do nothing to improve the metabolic reserve of bone tissue. In addition, just as I was writing this chapter, the FDA required two important new additions to the label warnings on all statin medications. The first is about a significant increase in blood glucose, glycosylated hemoglobin, and diabetes, and the other about "reversible" cognitive-related side effects such as memory loss or confusion. While these drugs may play a role in preventing certain outcomes, they do so by depleting the metabolic reserve of other critical physiological processes. There are over 30 million Americans taking a prescription statin drug.

ries. How about building up cartilage in the knee or antioxidants in the eyes that quench the free radicals that cause cataracts? This idea extends to nearly every system we could mention.

> *Building metabolic reserve through Lifestyle Synergy expands and even strengthens the buffers we will later rely upon to maintain our health. While it's never too late to begin building metabolic reserve, the earlier you start, the better.*

Chronic Disease and the Weakest Link

The great researcher Hans Selye, best known for his work in the area of physiological stress, once said, "*Among all my autopsies (and I have performed over 1000), I have never seen a person who died of old age. In fact, I do not think that anyone has ever died of old age yet. We invariably die because one vital part has worn out too early in proportion to the rest of the body.*" We might argue and say that people who die of old age rarely have autopsies performed upon them, but his point is still quite profound and important if we are to understand how chronic diseases are mediated and expressed in different tissues. We might say that chronic disease knows how to find the weakest link—or at least the canoe closest to the waterfall.

As researchers studying chronic diseases have discovered, there are common pathways that drive these dysfunctions—independent of the type of cell or tissue. Among these common pathways, the most frequently cited are inflammation and oxidation. These two pathways play a major role in obesity-related diseases, diabetes, cardiovascular disease, Alzheimer's disease, chronic kidney disease, arthritis, prostate disease, inflammatory bowel diseases, and nearly all cancers. While these two factors are responsible for depleting the metabolic reserve of critical tissues, the irony is that without inflammation or oxidation, we couldn't survive at all.

This is an important point. Unlike the acute diseases that mainly come from outside our bodies, chronic disease is almost always a result of "normal" processes wearing away our metabolic reserve and buffering capacity, even though these processes are designed to prevent them from becoming harmful. In most cases, it is the dysfunctions from within that allow the external threats to wreak their havoc, like the cold virus taking advantage of an immune system depleted of vital nutrients, or an innocent fall that leads to a hip fracture in a woman with depleted BMD. These external threats may have been rebuffed and even gone unnoticed but for the lack of metabolic reserve in these systems. The daily decisions we make that affect our metabolic reserve, whether good or bad, are helping to determine what area will be our weakest link.

To be fair, we must include two other factors that predispose and influence our risk for chronic disease. The first would be the genes we inherited from our parents; the second would be those environmental factors we cannot control. While these two factors are not insignificant, researchers still believe that 80–90% of most chronic diseases are preventable by proper lifestyle choices alone. In fact, lifestyle interventions can often change our genetic predisposition (something called epigenetics, which we will discuss in the next chapter) or trump genetic predisposition by altering gene expression. A great example of how lifestyle intervention can trump genetic predisposition was illustrated in one of the largest diabetes prevention studies called the Diabetes Prevention Program (DPP).[10]

The DPP study included over 3200 patients from twenty-seven different clinical centers throughout the U.S. All these patients were considered to be pre-diabetic because of their elevated fasting glucose and their impaired glucose tolerance as measured during an oral glucose tolerance test. The average baseline fasting glucose level in these patients was about 106 mg/dl (diabetes is diagnosed at 126 mg/dl); most were overweight or obese, with an average baseline BMI of 34 (73% of women and 56% of men met the criteria for obesity—a BMI > 30 kg/m^2). Each patient was assigned to one of three intervention groups: placebo, metformin therapy, or lifestyle intervention therapy.† Metformin was selected because in previous clinical trials this drug reduced the incidence of future diabetes in pre-diabetic patients.

---

† Something that is not well known about the DPP is that the study initially included a fourth intervention, troglitazone (Rezulin), which was discontinued from the study in 1998 because of the drug's potential liver toxicity, resulting in it being removed from the UK market late in 1997. Troglitazone was subsequently pulled from the U.S. market by the FDA in March of 2000. The data from this "4th arm" was not reported.

The lifestyle intervention group in the DPP had specific goals to reach. Patients were given frequent counseling sessions in order to help them lose 7% of their body weight in the first six months, with the goal to maintain that for four years; and they were to attempt to get 150 minutes of moderate physical activity per week, mostly in the form of walking.

All patients were followed for four years and tracked for changes in their weight, fasting blood glucose, glycosylated hemoglobin (a marker of long-term blood glucose control), and a number of other related health parameters. With much fanfare, the results of the first four years of the DPP trial, entitled "Reduction in the Incidence of Type 2 Diabetes with Lifestyle Intervention or Metformin," were published in the February 7, 2002 edition of the *New England Journal of Medicine.* The researchers found that within those four years, over 35% of patients given no intervention (placebo group) had developed type 2 diabetes; the average fasting blood glucose for this group rose gradually from 106 to almost 115 mg/dl—a continual stretching of the physiological resilience controlling blood sugar.

As you can see from Figure 5.4, metformin therapy lowered the cumulative incidence of type 2 diabetes by 31%, compared to the placebo

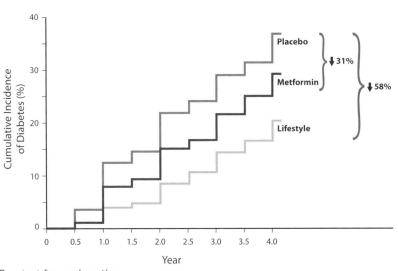

Figure 5.4 **Primary Outcome of Diabetes Prevention Program**

See text for explanation.

group. What surprised many, however, was the fact that the lifestyle intervention therapy nearly doubled this benefit, reducing the cumulative incidence of diabetes in that group by a full 58%. We don't have time to go into all the details here, but the lifestyle intervention group maintained this advantage of reduced diabetes incidence even ten years after beginning the trial and more than six years after the intervention ceased.[11] What I want to point out now is a study that was performed later, based on the genetic predisposition of the patients related to the outcomes of the DPP.

As it turns out, there are numerous genes, or gene variants, that are known to increase a person's risk for diabetes. By using thirty-four of the most common gene variants known to influence diabetes risk, researchers grouped all of the DPP participants into four groups based on their Genetic Risk Score (GRS) for diabetes.[12] What they found was quite fascinating. As one would expect, there was a statistical increase in diabetes incidence related to a higher GRS. However, in the group with the highest genetic risk (the 4th quartile of GRS), where the risk in the placebo group was highest, metformin therapy had virtually no impact at all (no statistical or clinical difference). Amazingly, when the highest GRS subjects were given lifestyle intervention, the diabetes incidence rate was just as low as in all the other genetic risk groups. At least in this study, these modest lifestyle changes seem to attenuate the increased risk due to genetic predisposition, something metformin could not accommodate. Lifestyle intervention was building up metabolic reserve and helping to prevent the metabolic drift toward diabetes. Drug intervention was unable to do this in patients with high genetic risk.

Unfortunately, this analysis is rarely seen by clinicians or patients. There are few people championing lifestyle interventions who have the time to go around and educate clinicians on the nuances related to genetic risk scores and diabetes incidence within the DPP. Actually, the opposite may be true. I recall attending the annual meeting of the American Diabetes Association the year following the publication of the original DPP trial. Walking through the vast array of booths touting the latest drugs, glucose monitors, and intervention strategies, I came across the booth of the company that sold the commercial brand of metformin—Glucophage. The data for the DPP trial was prominently displayed on numerous panels of their "booth," but someone in their graphics department had forgotten to include the information about the lifestyle intervention group on their graphs. They prominently showed the 31% reduction in risk from the metformin, but clinicians and nurses and diabetes educators would need to find out about the lifestyle intervention arm somewhere else. When would they ever have run across the data showing metformin had no effect in the patients with the highest genetic risk? Where would they find out that lifestyle medicine is nearly twice as powerful in its ability to reduce the incidence of diabetes than the drug they are being told to prescribe?

The Power of Lifestyle Synergy

In this chapter, we have only begun to define the mystery behind *vis medicatrix naturae,* the natural healing capacity of the body. We have outlined the basic mechanisms with which our bodies are designed to keep us healthy: rhythmic homeostasis, physiological resilience, and metabolic reserve. We even showed specific examples of how signals from our lifestyle choices are perfectly tailored to maintain our healing capacity while pharmaceuticals rarely perform this function.

To really understand how it all works, though, we will need to go one step further to open up the healing potential designed in our body. In order to truly understand the power driving the synergy produced by our lifestyle decisions and to keep up with where the future of medicine is heading, both the clinician and the patient will need to have some knowledge of a few slightly advanced topics: genetics, epigenetics, and genomics. In chapter 6 we will outline these important concepts in simple language and show why it is so important in our model, helping us explain, and even predict, a synergistic lifestyle intervention strategy.

CHAPTER 6

A Symphony of Signals

"The whole is greater than the sum of its parts."

—Aristotle (384 BC–322 BC)

IF YOU HAVE EVER had the opportunity to hear a world-class orchestra, you can appreciate how the synergy of thousands of single notes can transform into a fusion of symphonic sound. Likewise, when you begin to understand just a little about the marvelous and intricate inner workings of the cell, you will be just as amazed at both the simplicity and the complexity of how all those signals produce the health that sustains us. This chapter will explore those signals in a bit of detail and is one of the more important parts of this work if we are to really understand the power of lifestyle medicine and how our body is designed to convert lifestyle signals into health.[†] We will attempt to describe only the necessary elements of the signaling process, recognizing that there are other details that can impact the outcome that we won't cover here. We will leave those details for further study elsewhere.

[†] If you are tempted to skip this chapter because you think you won't understand these concepts or you just want to get to the "intervention" chapters, I would ask that you reconsider this strategy as you will miss the very heart of how and why each of the principles in those chapters works. If you are a clinician and you understand some of these concepts already, this chapter may help give you some ideas about how to describe these amazing concepts to those less familiar with them.

In the previous chapter, we laid out a number of basic concepts to describe how our bodies keep us healthy. One of those concepts was the notion of physiological resilience, the ability to compensate for poor signaling and to re-establish balance. In the current metabolic disease crisis, a system constantly being challenged is the one designed to maintain proper blood glucose. It is difficult to exaggerate the importance of maintaining proper blood glucose to avoid a wide range of chronic disease outcomes, and indispensable to that system is a very small protein hormone called insulin. Produced by specialized cells in the pancreas called beta cells, insulin is developed and secreted in response to increased blood sugar and provides a powerful signal to insulin-responsive cells, causing them to take glucose from the blood.

In general, the loss of blood sugar control that we call diabetes is basically a consequence of dysfunction in the insulin-producing pancreatic beta cells, resulting in insufficient insulin levels to move the glucose from the blood into the tissues. Type 1 diabetes (often called juvenile diabetes) results when these pancreatic beta cells are destroyed early in life by what appears to be an autoimmune self-destruction.[†] Type 2 diabetes (once called adult-onset diabetes) is generally a result of beta cell dysfunction brought about by the added stress placed upon the pancreatic beta cells in their attempt to produce ever-increasing amounts of insulin to compensate for a person's growing insulin resistance. Eventually, the stressed beta cells become dysfunctional and are destroyed, lowering the pancreas's insulin secretion and resulting in elevated blood glucose.

But if insulin is so important to control blood glucose, why don't the liver or the kidneys, or any other tissue for that matter, start producing insulin? After all, every cell in our body has the insulin gene. In fact, we could ask this question for literally thousands of processes that are occurring every second in our bodies. What makes one type of cell function in a completely different way than the thousands of other cells in our body? What causes the beta cells to produce insulin in response to

---

† The exact cause of type 1 diabetes is debated. It appears there may be several different insults that can occur throughout life (most typically in early life) that can trigger a rapid onset of beta cell destruction thought to be mediated by autoimmune processes, leading to the failure to produce insulin.

rising blood glucose levels and the nearby alpha cells of the pancreas to produce the counter-regulatory hormone glucagon in response to low blood sugar? If all our cells have the same DNA and the same genes, how is it possible that each type of cell performs radically different roles in the human body? The answer to these questions is one of the most fascinating findings of the past few decades.

Figure 6.1 **The Same DNA Produces a Diversity of Cells**

Different Cell Types

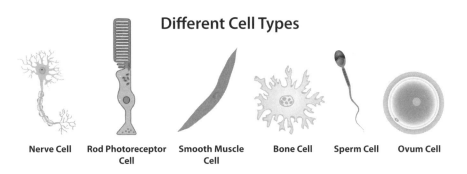

| Nerve Cell | Rod Photoreceptor Cell | Smooth Muscle Cell | Bone Cell | Sperm Cell | Ovum Cell |

The size, shape and function of the 200 or so different types of cells that make up our bodies each have the exact same DNA. It is clear that the outcome of cellular function is determined by gene expression, not DNA sequence alone. Note: Relative size of cells not shown.

Gazing into a mirror, it is hard to believe that we all started out as one single cell, receiving half of our genetic material from each parent at the point of conception. The information that would drive who we would become, for the most part, is encoded in the forty-six strands of DNA (chromosomes) that we received on that auspicious occasion. From that original, undifferentiated single cell we have now multiplied to over 50 trillion cells, distributed into at least 200 distinct cell types. Those twenty-three chromosomal pairs hold your genetic and health *potential*, but, as we will soon show, they do not always determine your health *outcome*.

If we think of each chromosome as a cookbook containing thousands of recipes (genes), we might say, by way of analogy, that we have 46 cookbooks in our library. The *potential* for thousands of different recipes, like having 46 different cookbooks in your kitchen, doesn't necessarily tell us what we will be having for supper. So it is with each cell. Even though every cell has the same genetic information, the genes expressed in each cell (i.e. which recipes are used) will differ depending on the cell type, the stage of embryonic development, and the consequences of a host of cell-signaling events. Developmental biology tells us that the single cell, formed as the product of conception, is pluripotent, which means it has the potential to become any type of cell. With each cell division, an imprinted set of signals causes the growing number of cells to differentiate, expressing certain genes and silencing others. In the end, the characteristics that define each cell are not determined by genetics per se, since they all have the same DNA, but instead by genetic expression. Said another way: each cell has the same set of cookbooks, but they are reading different pages and making different recipes.

The Central Dogma of Gene Expression

Figure 6.2 **How Genes Become Proteins and Control Cell Function**

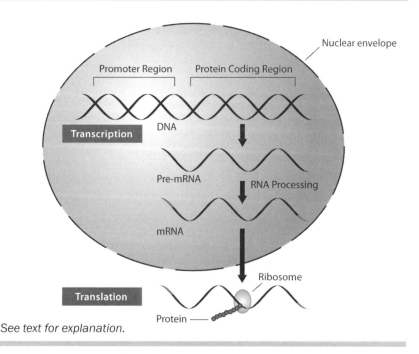

See text for explanation.

In case you have forgotten the basics of genetic expression, here is a quick primer of the central dogma of biology. Our cells hold genetic information in their nucleus as three billion base pairs of DNA (on forty-six separate strands we call chromosomes). Within the double-stranded DNA molecule are sections of protein-encoding sequences we call "genes," as well as numerous other regulatory sequences once thought of as "junk" DNA. The "Central Dogma" of biology generally describes how the information encoded in our DNA is converted into the proteins that give our bodies function and then, in turn, protect the information stored within the strands of DNA (See Figure 6.2).

Basically, in order for a gene to be expressed as a protein it must first have its protein-encoding information converted into a single strand of RNA called messenger RNA (mRNA) in a process known as transcription. Along the DNA strand there is a region next to the protein-encoding sequence known as the promoter region. This portion of the gene allows for the attachment of several proteins, including RNA polymerase, which is then responsible for creating the mRNA as a virtual copy of the protein-encoding gene. As we will see later, access to the promoter-region of a gene controls gene expression. Once this mRNA strand is processed, it is transported out of the nucleus into the cytoplasm of the cell, where the information in the coding sequence of this mRNA is translated into a string of amino acids to create a protein. This process of translating mRNA into protein is performed by ribosomes, complexes of proteins and special ribosomal RNA molecules. The translated proteins might go on to become structural components of the cell or extracellular matrix, enzymes for metabolic reactions, hormones (like insulin), and hundreds of other cell-signaling molecules. The intricate and tight regulation of the conversion of information from DNA into protein is the heart of how lifestyle signals are translated into health.

Good Genes, Bad Genes

Of course, we know that there is a wide range of subtle differences within gene sequences in the human populations, a variety of genotypes (gene sequences) and phenotypes (physical characteristics). The most obvious are those that affect our hair and eye color, but there are numerous differences in genes that are quite a bit less obvious. Even within our own genome we might have two different variations of the same gene, a different one from each parent. If we inherit two identical genes from each parent, it is said that we are homozygous for that gene; if we inherit two different genes, we are heterozygous for that gene. In the case of heterozygous genes, if each gene encodes a slightly different protein with different characteristics or, in the case of enzymes, different activity levels, our phenotype or metabolism is often a blend of the characteristics of these two genes. If one or both genes are defective, severe genetic disorders can occur.

Since the historic Human Genome Project deciphered the DNA sequence of humans, we can now "read" the DNA sequence of each gene. What we have discovered is that there are a lot more subtle differences between genes than we once thought. In fact, there are many genes that differ by just one single base pair, called single nucleotide polymorphisms (SNPs or "snips"). In a gene sequence that is perhaps thousands of base pairs long, how could one single base pair change the outcome of gene expression? Sometimes, just one base pair will result in a change in the mRNA stability, reducing the level of translatable messages and expressed proteins or simply changing a single amino acid along the protein sequence. Depending on which amino acid is impacted, a range of altered activities may affect the function of the expressed protein. Using modern molecular biology techniques, researchers and clinicians can easily measure a person's DNA sequence, looking for SNPs known to affect our health. We will look at just one example.

One of the best-characterized SNPs is located in the gene that expresses a protein that helps to convert folic acid into its active biological molecule, methyltetrahydrofolate. The protein is abbreviated as MTHFR, which stands for methylenetetrahydrofolate reductase; the gene that encodes this protein is the *MTHFR* gene. In sequencing the gene, researchers discovered that some individuals had a cytosine (C) at base pair position 677 (this is the most common), and others had thymidine (T) at that position. This is often referred to as *MTHFR* C677T polymorphism and causes an alanine to valine amino acid change at the 222 position of the protein. This small change in the protein actually alters its characteristics, resulting in less efficient synthesis of active folate compounds. Most individuals in the U.S. are homozygous for the normal variant (677CC), but up to 10% of the population may be homozygous for the other variant (677TT). These individuals often have noticeably less efficient methylation, accounting for higher risk for certain diseases and a higher need for dietary folate consumption or folic acid supplementation.

Epigenetics: Going Above and Beyond

What we all learned in high school about heredity and genetics is being turned on its head by the emerging science called epigenetics (epi- in Greek means "above" or "upon"). If the classic understanding of genetics explains how cells can replicate their DNA sequence, passing along that sequence through cell division, epigenetics describes the heritable genetic changes that occur without ever changing the DNA sequence. Epigenetics, in simple terms, is a series of chemical tags attached to the DNA sequence (or the proteins upon which DNA winds itself) that can influence genetic expression in the cell. If genetics defines the recipes in the cookbooks, then epigenetics is like placing bookmarks or folding the "ears" down to make particular recipes easier to find; or conversely, dripping maple syrup on a page to stick two pages together, making those recipes harder to find. Science has now discovered that we inherit from our parents and accumulate over our lifetimes epigenetic changes that influence gene expression, determine our need for specific nutrients, and impact our risk for various chronic diseases.

Without getting into too many details, epigenetic influences occur by three basic mechanisms: DNA methylation, histone modification, and production of microRNA (miRNA) sequences (see Figure 6.3).[†] DNA methylation is the most straightforward, and it describes the attachment of a methyl-group onto one of the base pairs that make up the strand of DNA. When DNA is methylated, especially in the promoter region, it can inhibit the genetic expression protein complex from binding, effectively repressing (silencing) the expression of that gene. There is ample evidence that hyper-methylation or hypo-methylation can result in aberrant gene expression, leading to various chronic diseases.

---

† These are the three mechanisms we know about today. It would not surprise me if we discover more epigenetic mechanisms in the near future.

Figure 6.3 **The Mechanisms of Epigenetics**

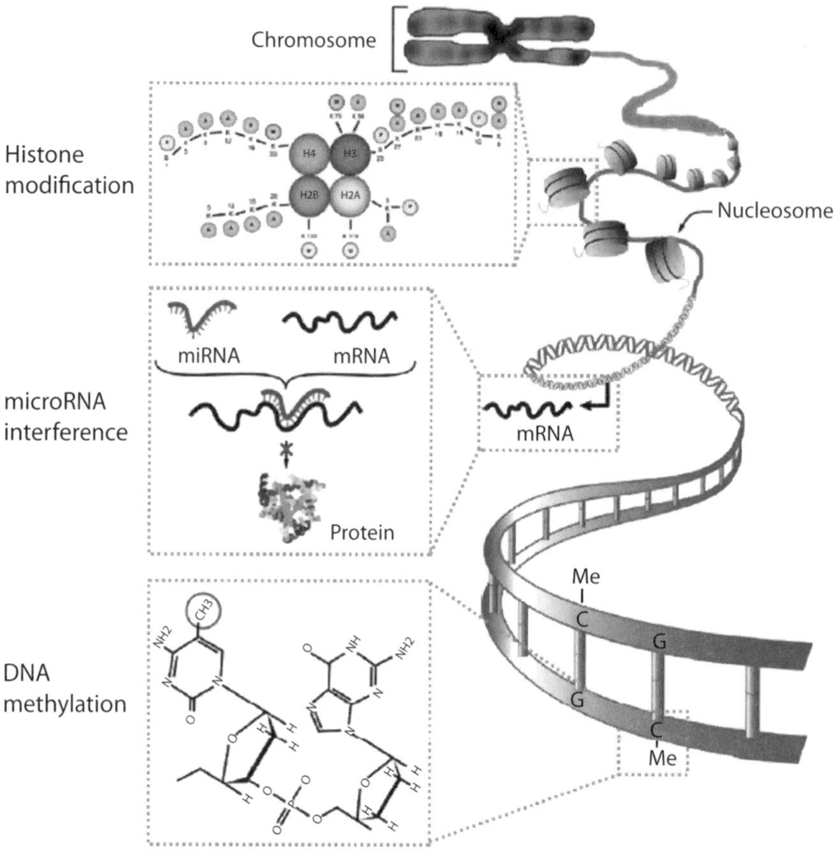

Histone modification

microRNA interference

DNA methylation

Chromosome

Nucleosome

miRNA   mRNA

mRNA

Protein

Me

C

G

G

C

Me

See Text for explanation.   Adapted from reference 20- with permission.

Since the three million base pairs of DNA in each cell's nucleus would be impossible to manage if it were all unwound, like an unwieldy garden hose, DNA is packaged into a complex called chromatin, like tightly-wrapped "beads on a string." The string is the DNA itself and the beads are a set of proteins called histones that act to wind up and package each long strand of DNA into a manageable volume. While this packaging of DNA is great for managing the space consumed by each chromosome, it essentially keeps most of the genes hidden from the protein machinery that translates genes into mRNA molecules. Determining which area of the genome is available for gene expression is greatly influenced by the actions of the histones. The second mechanism that allows for epigenetic changes is histone modification, which describes specific biochemical modifications made to the histone proteins themselves. Certain tags (like methylation, acetylation, phosphorylation, etc.) enable these histones to open up, allowing certain genes to be accessible to the cell's gene expression machinery, while others cause the histones to close up, preventing other genes from becoming accessible to the gene expression machinery.

Lastly, the recent discovery of microRNA explains how yet another mechanism influences gene expression without changing the DNA sequence itself. Since gene expression requires that the DNA-to-protein conversion maintains a stable mRNA signal (not to be confused with miRNA), anything that destabilizes or counteracts the mRNA signal will influence gene expression and cellular function. MicroRNAs are small sequences of RNA that can bind to mRNA sequences, hindering their ability to be translated into protein (the process is technically called post-transcriptional repression). Scientists now believe that perhaps 1000 different miRNA sequences, unknown before the 1990s, are encoded in the human genome, influencing the expression of up to 60% of our genes.[1] †A flurry of research over just the past few years has uncovered numerous influences of specific miRNA sequences and chronic disease pathways, including research into ways to modify miRNA to prevent or treat chronic diseases.[2,3]

Now you might be saying to yourself, "That's just about all the molecular biology I want to know for now." I hear you, so let's move to a brief discussion about why this matters. As we said before, our DNA sequence might play a major role in who we become, but gene expression translates the potential of our DNA into health or disease. It is not nature versus nurture, but nature being acted upon by nurture. More importantly, while we have virtually no control over our DNA sequence, we have numerous ways to influence our gene expression. In the case of epigenetic changes, these influences can stay with us for a

---

† A recent study has revealed that by injecting specific cardiac cell miRNA into fibroblasts (skin-like cells), the genetic expression and metabolic machinery were completely reprogrammed into that of a cardiac muscle cell. The implications for this type of research for repairing damaged tissue are enormous and reveal the influence of DNA sequences previously called "junk" DNA.

while since they are passed on as cells divide and can even be passed on to future generations if these changes influence the DNA in our germ cells (sperm or egg cells).

The classic animal model that describes the power of epigenetic influence is the agouti mouse model.[4] This particular strain of mice has a genetic susceptibility to become obese, which also corresponds to a change in coat color (yellow or agouti). This genetic susceptibility appeared to be defined by classic genetic mechanisms since it was easily passed on from one generation of mice to another. It wasn't until Randy Jirtle, Ph.D., a researcher at Duke University, and his colleagues fed female agouti mice a diet that increases DNA methylation before and during pregnancy that they discovered something unexpected. Agouti mice born to mothers fed a diet rich in methyl donors were brown instead of yellow, thin instead of obese. The expression of the agouti gene was silenced when the DNA of the mother's egg cell was properly methylated, passing a "silenced" gene to her offspring. The gene was there, but the gene expression was not. The epigenetic genie was out of the bottle, and it will forever change how we understand heritable traits.

But it's not just mothers who can affect these epigenetic patterns. Fathers can also pass along hereditary tags to their offspring as well. The seminal paper that described this was published in *Nature* in 2010.[5] Researchers showed that male rats fed a high-fat diet passed along epigenetically tagged DNA to their offspring that resulted in early beta-cell dysfunction, insulin resistance, and obesity. They linked the high-fat diet with reduced methylation, which altered the expression of over 2000 different genes. What is even more disturbing is that other factors may add, in a synergistic fashion, to the negative imprinting of our genetic expression. We see this in animal studies showing that when the toxic compound Bisphenol A (BPA) is given to pregnant animals along with a high-fat diet, it creates a heritable and negative metabolic consequence in their offspring.[6] (We will have more to say about BPA and other environmental influences in chapter 12.)

Of course, there is some good news here. Scientists are publishing on a regular basis reports describing how various compounds from food can positively impact gene expression through epigenetic mechanisms, either on a permanent or a temporary basis. One of the most well-known of these relationships is the importance of methyl donors during pregnancy; the most commonly described is the need for folate (folic acid) supplementation even before conception. Since appropriate methylation is one of the key factors that determines proper cell-specific gene expression throughout life, maintaining a diet with a balance of methyl donors is critical.[7] †

It is my belief that over the last two centuries or more, epigenetic changes have been accumulating from generation to generation, accounting for the compounded chronic disease crisis we are currently experiencing. In the river of life, each generation is starting off farther downstream, sometimes with a hole in their paddle. Even so, the capacity of our cells to receive signals from our lifestyle decisions is still large enough to overcome most of our genetic and epigenetic ancestry. We will move to that discussion now.

Cell Signaling: The Basics

Now that we know why one cell is different from another, based mostly upon which genes are silent and which genes are "turned on," let us explore the whole cell more closely. Figure 6.4 shows a generic cell, with its outer cell membrane defining the size and shape of the cell itself. The membrane is made of a lipid bilayer (phospholipids and cholesterol) that is embedded with thousands of different proteins. The membrane acts to separate the cytoplasm of the cell from the extracellular matrix and is the communication center between the cell and the outside world. Within the cytoplasm are thousands of proteins and metabolites that are performing the functional tasks of the cell in a highly coordinated fashion. Organelles, separated by their own membranes, are also located within the cytoplasm with their special tasks: the nucleus housing the genetic information, the mitochondria producing energy (ATP) for the cell, the endoplasmic reticulum helping to package our proteins and lipids, and many other organelles involved with transporting proteins or waste materials throughout the cell.

---

† Basic dietary components that improve methylation would be methionine, choline, folic acid/folates, vitamin B12, and vitamin B6. Supplements containing these as well as Betaine (Trimethylglycine-TMG), S-Adenosylmethionine (SAM), or Methylsulfonylmethane (MSM) have all been used successfully to improve methylation in humans.

For our purpose here, we want to discuss how signals from either inside or outside the cell, even signals from inside and outside the body, influence gene expression and cell function. We will start with one that is relevant to our discussion—the impact of insulin upon a cell. As it turns out, glucose from the blood or tissue doesn't just diffuse into cells. In fact, since most body fluids are water-soluble, the lipid bilayer of the cell membrane prevents most metabolites from passively entering the cell. Instead, cells have glucose transporters that act like little tunnels or pores to allow glucose to enter the cell.

Obviously, this pore can't be available and open all the time in all cells, because this would lead to an unregulated and constant depletion of blood glucose as well as high intracellular glucose, even when the cell doesn't need it for energy. Instead, the cell keeps special glucose transporters sequestered in small membrane rafts, or vesicles, that are kept away from the cell surface, ready to be deployed if they are called into action. When the blood sugar rises and the pancreas produces and secretes insulin, the insulin molecule eventually makes its way to the cell, perhaps a fat cell around your waist. When that insulin molecule binds to the insulin receptor of the cell, a chain of chemical reactions occurs (in this case, phosphorylation reactions) in a split second that leads to thousands of different outcomes in the cell. We call these chemical reactions cell signaling, and in this case, insulin signaling. Like a series of dominos falling, or a baton being handed from one protein to another, the original insulin signals result in the translocation of our glucose transporters to the cell surface, where they then merge with the cell membrane, allowing glucose to come into the cell. Each cell in our body receives hundreds or thousands of similar signals each and every day, signaling and coordinating every minutia of our metabolic machinery.

Besides the insulin-dependent glucose transport signal, other signals driven by insulin-binding cause specific proteins from the cytoplasm to migrate into the nucleus, turning on the specific gene expression to create proteins that help metabolize glucose into energy, or in the case of our fat cell, maybe to convert extra glucose into fatty acids. One signal, in this case insulin, can have a major impact upon thousands of different activities in the cell.

Figure 6.4 **Glucose Transport via Insulin Signaling**

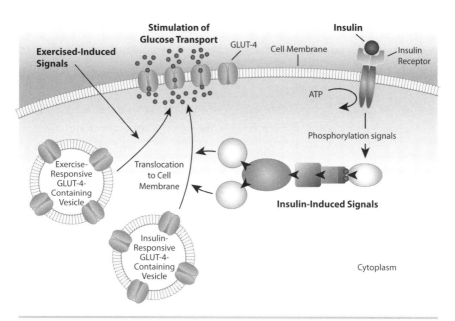

When insulin binds to the insulin receptor, a cascade of chemical signals (through many different proteins) eventually causes GLUT4 containing vesicles to translocate to the cell membrane where they can allow glucose to enter the cell. In muscle cells, GLUT4 containing vesicle also respond to signals induced by exercise- independent of insulin.

Genomics and Other "Omics"

Now that we have gotten our feet wet with some understanding of genetics, epigenetics, and cell signaling, we need to discuss some technical terms being thrown around quite a bit in medical circles these days. The term "genomics" describes the influence of a person's genome (all genetic material) on their health. But since we know that all genetic material doesn't turn into mRNA transcripts or proteins or end up affecting metabolites, we now have terms to describe these influences as well. When we add this terminology to the agents that influence them, we get yet another layer of terminology. So, for instance, the study of nutrients that influence genetic expression is now called nutritional genomics or nutrigenomics.[†] These terms were virtually unknown just a few decades ago, but today they are the buzz at nearly every scientific and medical conference.

Currently, any substance thought to influence health (positively or negatively) will be tested in cell culture or animal or human studies to see what influence it has upon the total mRNA expression (called the transcriptome), the pattern of proteins expressed (proteome), and the resulting metabolites (metabolome) of the cell (see Figure 6.5). In fact, nowadays scientists routinely screen thousands of natural substances, looking for changes in the transcriptome or proteome of different tissues or cells with which the substance has been incubated. When they find that a substance significantly increases or decreases specific transcripts, proteins, or metabolites, they can follow this with more specific studies to decipher the relationship or mechanism.

Figure 6.5 **The Language of the Basic Levels of Genomics**

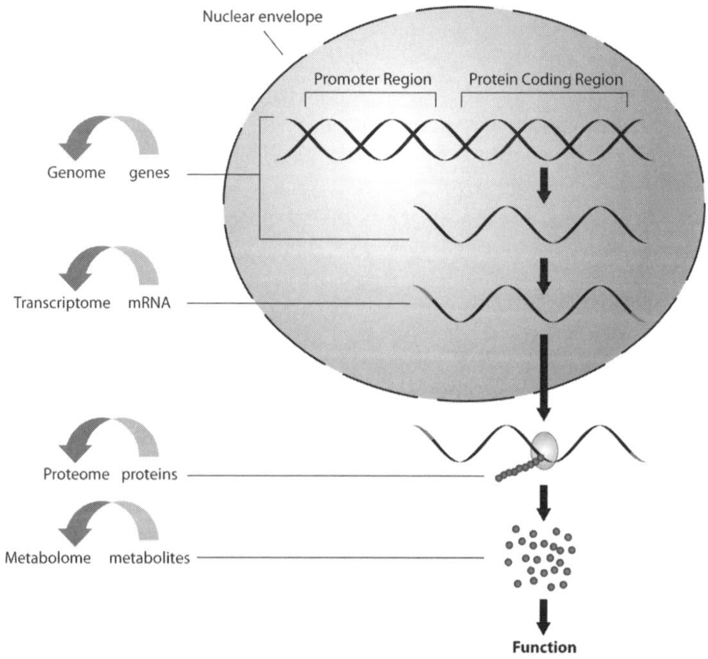

[†] There is literally no end to the combination of terms in the "omic" field. We have epigenomics, nutriproteinomics, nutrimetabolomics, as well as others we will see later.

An Apple a Day

With this in mind, we can now start talking about all those "signals" we have been alluding to thus far. To break this down a little bit, we will use a familiar friend, the apple. We have all heard the old adage "an apple a day keeps the doctor away," and epidemiology appears to back up this notion. In fact, data collected in a number of different cohorts has shown that people who frequently eat apples are at reduced risk for lung and colon cancer, asthma and COPD, cardiovascular disease, Alzheimer's disease, and type 2 diabetes.[8-10] And these are just the conditions for which we have definitive evidence so far. How can one single food be so powerful? Let's consider the many signals provided by this humble fruit.

The average-sized apple (with the skin) weighs about 185 grams (6.4 oz.). It contains

- 156 grams of water (water in food accounts for about 20% of our total intake).
- 25 grams of carbohydrates, 19 of that as sugar.
- 4.4 grams of fiber to slow the absorption of sugar, which reduces the glycemic impact of the sugar itself. Fiber also improves the "microbiome," which describes the living microorganisms in our colon.
- Very little protein and a small amount (0.4 grams) of fat.
- Low to modest levels of numerous vitamins (A, C, E, K, B1, B2, B3, B5, B6, and folate) and minerals (calcium, magnesium, iron, potassium, and phosphorus)
- Dozens of plant compounds called phytonutrients such as carotenoids, flavonoids, and organic acids.[†]

Just in this brief survey alone, we can see that our medium apple, eaten with the skin, has the capacity to deliver at least a few dozen signals, most of which have been shown to improve our health. Mash it up as apple sauce and you diminish the fiber content; make it into apple

---

† Certain varieties of apples have a higher content of polyphenols; the highest are Fuji, Red Delicious, Gala, Liberty, Northern Spy, and Golden Delicious.

juice and you have now processed our wonderful apple into a high gly-cemic-index drink, very different from the low glycemic-impact signals provided by the whole fruit. Remove the skin and you lose a number of those important vitamins and phytonutrients; but if you purchase com-mercial apples and don't wash the skin, you might be adding signals from harmful agricultural chemicals. Can an apple be this complicated? Permit me to take this one step further as we look at the signaling ca-pacity and health benefits of just one particular phytonutrient found in the skin of apples.

There is a class of polyphenolic compounds called flavonoids that make up a large portion of the phytonutrients in an apple, and among the flavonoids present in apples we will focus our attention on querce-tin.[†] Perhaps one of the most studied plant flavonoids, quercetin has been shown to have numerous health-promoting functions in most mammalian systems, including humans.[11] I would love to spend the time listing the thousands of studies here for you (textbooks have been written about the health benefits of flavonoids), but I will leave that to the most ambitious readers to look up for themselves.[12,13] I will stick with just a few studies to show you the power of the nutrigenomic influ-ence of quercetin.

Recall the genomic influence of the high-fat diet we mentioned above. This model is often used in animal studies to show how poor di-etary patterns can influence gene expression, because it typically leads to all the abnormalities of insulin resistance, fatty liver disease, dyslipid-emia, cardiovascular disease, and oxidative damage that are so often seen in individuals consuming a human version of this diet. We have already shown that a high-fat diet can cause hereditary influences in the offspring of animals consuming this diet, but once these influences are inherited, can the offspring do anything to change this pattern of gene expression?

By feeding rats a high-fat diet, researchers can measure changes in the gene expression (transcriptome) and protein levels (proteome) of important genes and proteins regulating lipid metabolism and related

---

† Actually, there are several quercetin conjugates found in the skin of the apple like quer-cetin-3-galactoside, quercetin-3-glucoside, and quercetin-3-rhamnoside. Quercetin con-jugates are found in many fruits, vegetables, and plants, especially apples, yellow onions, citrus fruits, and green tea.

physiological outcomes. When these same animals are given a high-fat diet along with dietary levels of quercetin, they are able to reverse those changes in gene expression and protein synthesis, virtually eliminating the physiological changes leading to lipid abnormalities, fatty accumulation in the liver, and accumulation of body fat in these animals.[14] Essentially, adding quercetin to the diet in these animals blunted much of the negative impact by altering which genes were turned on and which were turned off. Here we have one positive signal (quercetin) competing with several negative signals (high-fat diet), showing how powerful a single molecule like quercetin can be. In fact, other researchers have shown (using a different animal model) that quercetin can influence the expression of well over 2000 different genes, depending on the concentration present in the cell.[15] It is no wonder that epidemiologists continue to show that the health risk for nearly every chronic disease is lower in those who consume sufficient flavonoids.[15-19] The standard American diet is woefully deficient in flavonoid consumption.

Quercetin and related flavonoids are now frequently used as dietary supplements (capsules, tablets, and powders) and have been tested in clinical trials as antioxidants, immune modulators; and for anti-viral, anti-hypertensive, and anti-inflammatory functions; exercise recovery; endothelial function; and lipid metabolism, to name just a few. I am a strong advocate for the consumption of quercetin from dietary and dietary-supplement sources. Over the years, I have developed no less than a dozen products using quercetin to support a wide range of clinical conditions.

Now imagine if we looked at all the other phytonutrients in the apple. How many more nutrigenomic signals would we find? Now add to this oranges, broccoli, tomatoes, spinach, berries, and every other vegetable, fruit, and spice and you get an idea of how many potential signals can be derived from our diet alone. Food is information. Some of that information comes into the body (glucose) and then triggers secondary signals with great systemic impact (insulin). Other times, those signals go directly to the cells (phytonutrients), where they act as chemical modulators (antioxidant) or gene regulators (genomic signaling). You can now see why I believe that one of the keys to the metabolic disease crisis we are experiencing is a direct result of a change in lifestyle signals. Any change in dietary habits that diminishes the diversity of the foods we consume might result in the removal of thousands of phytonutrients that help signal how our cells modulate their metabolism.

When it comes to understanding the signals that explain how our lifestyle affects our health, diet is the first thing that comes to mind. We can take a food, like the apple, and analyze each chemical component, then turn around and test those isolated components in cell culture and animal models. But diet and dietary components are just one set of signals that our cells use to promote our health. We also mentioned above how Bisphenol A, a toxin, can mimic some of the same changes in gene expression as those of a high-fat diet, and we also mentioned insulin, which responds to food signals, but there are many more we haven't discussed. Some of these signals come to the cells in a monthly rhythm, like the hormones estrogen and progesterone in a premenopausal woman; others might come suddenly, like the inflammatory signals sent out by our immune cells after breathing in cigarette smoke. One of the most powerful signals, the last one we will discuss here, comes from the way our brain perceives the world around us.

Are You on Steroids?

Waking up in the morning is a "stressful" experience, or at least our body appears to think so. In fact, within the first thirty minutes of arising in the morning our body will produce its highest levels of the stress hormone cortisol. Perhaps you have been prescribed one of its pharmaceutical cousins in the form of cortisone, hydrocortisone, or prednisone as a potent steroid anti-inflammatory drug. If so, you know how powerful the effect of corticosteroids can be, both in their benefits and in their side effects. As it turns out, the cortisol produced in our bodies in response to stress has the same potent effects.

Since we will cover the ways in which cortisol is stimulated by stress in another chapter, I want to limit our discussion here to the way in which cortisol acts as an internal signal, directly impacting cell function. Figure 6.6 below shows a simplified diagram of cortisol signaling. Unlike insulin, which stays outside the cell, only binding to a membrane receptor, cortisol is transported into the cell cytoplasm where it can bind directly to a protein called the cortisol or glucocorticoid receptor (GR). The availability of the free cortisol that reaches the cytoplasm and eventually binds to the GR is controlled by a number of factors, which we won't discuss here, that can be influenced by signals from both inside and outside our body.

Figure 6.6 **How Cortisol Changes Gene Expression**

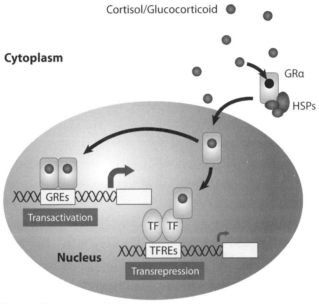

See Text for details.

Once cortisol binds to its receptor in the cytoplasm, this complex is transported into the nucleus. A group of proteins called heat shock proteins (HSPs) keep the GR from migrating prematurely into the nucleus. These HSPs are released when cortisol binds the GR, allowing the cortisol–GR complex to move into the nucleus. Once inside the nucleus, there are two potential actions that can result: activation (turning on) or repression (turning off) of gene expression. In the promoter region of certain genes is a sequence called a glucocorticoid response element (GRE) that permits the cortisol-bound GR to bind to it. Once bound, the GRE can recruit the other necessary proteins required for gene expression, initiating the mRNA transcript needed to later translate proteins we could describe as "cortisol-induced." Conversely, our cortisol-bound GR also can interfere with expression of other genes by binding to transcription factors already attached to the promoter region of those other genes. Like putting handcuffs on a juggler, the efficiency of the gene expression is diminished greatly. Like insulin, cortisol is another great example of how a single signal can modulate a number of gene families in a coordinated fashion, the outcome of which we might call the global cortisol response. Since every cell has the same DNA, the cortisol response in each is determined by epigenetic tags (not all genes are available in every cell), time of day (cortisol fluctuates throughout the day), and any other signals that influence the expression of the genes that coordinate the cortisol response. Mindboggling, yes; but simply amazing when you really think about it.

The Symphony of Signals

This brief discussion of genetics, epigenetics, and cell signaling can be both overwhelming and awe-inspiring. Like listening to a massive orchestra where hundreds of musicians blend their sounds together to produce a symphony, sometimes it is difficult to pick out a single instrument or figure out how the sounds of the brass instruments blend so effortlessly with the strings. When you are familiar with a piece of music, you can learn to hear the nuances that you never realized were there, and your appreciation for the piece is enhanced. If you could see all the score sheets for each instrument, you would realize that the symphony is merely the coordinated efforts of thousands of single notes played at the right time by hundreds of different, individual instruments. One or two sounds out of tune or out of time, and the whole symphony suffers.

Believe it or not, we have just scratched the surface of this massive topic, though I think you now have a basic foundation. To say that epigenetics and genomics are the research of the future is a gross understatement. Nearly every discipline of biology and medicine is employing these techniques and methods to understand how signals (food, drugs, sunlight, sleep, toxins) impact the cellular response. If we are to leverage the signals embedded in our lifestyle decisions, we must employ this knowledge as well. We will continue to refer to these ideas as we explore the principles and proofs of the Lifestyle Synergy Model throughout the rest of the book.

CHAPTER 7

Leveraging Lifestyle as Intervention

---

*"Policies are many, principles are few;
policies will change, principles never do."*

—John Maxwell (1947–)

IN THE PREVIOUS CHAPTERS, we have shown, in a wide array of mechanistic detail, how the overlapping systems keeping us healthy are intricately designed. By combining hundreds and thousands of signals, each cell responds in a highly coordinated fashion to produce the necessary proteins, metabolites, and additional messenger molecules that maintain signaling pathways going to other cells and tissues within the cascade of mechanisms that make us function properly. Although it's true that the power of the lifestyle decisions driving our health comes from the synergy of those many different signals, it is often difficult to know where one set of lifestyle signals ends and another begins. So while our ultimate recommendation is that "lifestyle" should be viewed as a cohesive and synergistic whole, we will need to unpack the concept into some traditional categories in order to evaluate the evidence and make specific recommendations. We know, for instance, that just telling people to "live healthier" is unlikely to influence their behavior. It is simply too vague, lacking any sort of specifics that can be implemented.

Even clinicians who hear about "lifestyle" as part of a healthy thera-peutic strategy are often at a loss when it comes to giving their patients specific recommendations, even though the official guideline recom-mendation for most chronic diseases includes lifestyle intervention as the foundation for all treatment protocols.[†] According to the 2000 Na-tional Health Interview Survey (NHIS), fewer than one in four respon-dents say they received any physician advice on either diet or exercise. High-risk patients often have a slightly higher chance of getting some advice from their clinician, although this advice is rarely tied to the patient's lifestyle habits (good or bad), nor followed by specific recom-mendations or programs to implement, both of which are critical for success. Research suggests that when obese individuals are advised to lose weight by their clinician, less than 20% of the time is that advice accompanied by a specific plan, even though studies suggest that obese patients who are given a plan (rather than merely advice) are five times more likely to achieve key objectives in their physical activity and di-etary goals.[1,2] Even when a plan is offered, rarely does it extend beyond diet and exercise; and while these are critical components of any life-style intervention program (as we will outline in some detail), much more is necessary if we are to use the synergy of lifestyle inputs to ef-fectively combat the current paradigm driving chronic disease.

Our first step, then, is to define the seven spheres or categories of the Lifestyle Synergy Model—each with discrete boundaries, more or less. I say more or less because many of these spheres are related to and dependent upon signals that come from one or more of the other spheres. The inter-related nature of the spheres is not only inevitable, since research has not fully defined all lifestyle signals independently, but actually part of what generates much of the synergy within the sys-tem itself. Now let's look at the seven spheres.

[†] Of particular note are the JNC guidelines for pre-hypertension and hypertension, the NCEP ATP guidelines for reducing risk based on cholesterol and lipid-related disorders, and the ADA's guidelines for treating both diabetic and pre-diabetic patients—but this is true of almost every official guideline panel making recommendations for chronic disease around the globe.

The Seven Spheres of the Lifestyle Synergy Model

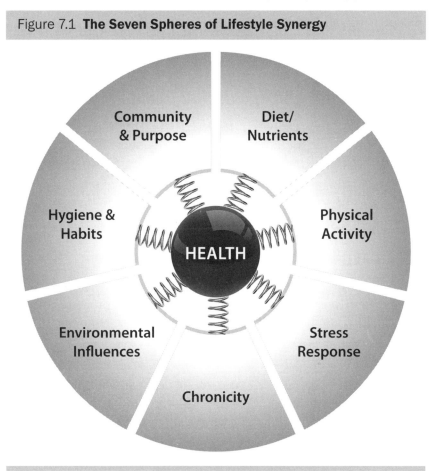

Figure 7.1 **The Seven Spheres of Lifestyle Synergy**

Community & Purpose

Diet/ Nutrients

Hygiene & Habits

Physical Activity

HEALTH

Environmental Influences

Stress Response

Chronicity

Diet and Nutrition:

When we think of lifestyle intervention, diet and nutrition are usually the first things to come to mind. Not surprisingly, there is more data on the health consequences of various diet options and food selections than all the other spheres combined, especially if you add all the studies on dietary supplements. While this sphere includes the obvious dietary choices and eating patterns, it also includes other things such as cooking styles, eating habits, and eating frequency. Of course, what we drink is included as well. Chapter 8 will lay out the research trends defining how dietary choices affect chronic disease outcomes as well as some of what we know about using dietary changes as an intervention tool. We will also lay out dietary principles that you can use to develop a personal or professional strategy to leverage your dietary habits within the broader context of maintaining your health.

Physical Activity:

Probably the second most popular form of lifestyle intervention, often coupled with diet, would be physical activity, mostly in the form of exercise. But we must think of physical activity as much more than just exercise; physical activity includes all our movements—even our non-activities, like being sedentary. Within the principle of physical activity outlined in chapter 9 we include postural habits, flexibility, and proper spinal alignment.

Stress and the Stress Response:

Our mental and emotional health is vital if we are to maximally leverage lifestyle medicine. The part of our brain that processes the perception of mental and emotional stress (the hypothalamus) is also the key to managing nearly every other important system of our bodies (glucose regulation, satiety, blood pressure, thyroid function, growth signaling, reproduction, etc.). We will devote a significant amount of time in chapter 10 to show how important the stress response system is when it comes to maintaining our health and how we can improve the buffering capacity of this important sphere of the Lifestyle Synergy Model.

Chronicity:

There is a growing scientific field called chronobiology, which studies how biological systems (plants and animals—including humans) are tightly regulated based on various intervals of time. The daily circadian rhythm is the most widely studied. Our body's chronicity (or lack thereof) has a great influence on the previous sphere in that the hypothalamus is part of the regulatory mechanisms keeping our internal clock working. The most researched component of this sphere is sleep, and we will focus much of our discussion on this most important "reset button" of our physiology. We will also discuss the role of weekly, monthly, yearly, and even lifetime cycles to show that as we move away from those external signals (the things that keep our internal clock in sync) we drift away from a healthy pattern of living. You can set your watch by the principles laid out in chapter 11.

Environmental Influences:

Often when we think about environmental influences we are conditioned to think only about negative environmental signals, things such as toxins from our air or water or radiation from electromagnetic fields. More broadly, however, we want to discuss how our body interacts with the environment, receiving a host of signals, good and bad. Obviously, we will discuss how toxins from our environment can adversely affect our health, but our environment includes so many wonderful signals: sunlight, air, temperature fluctuations, music, and the aesthetic beauty of nature. Sure, the healing process might at times require the four walls of a hospital room, but it might also be facilitated by sitting next to a brook, listening to the water jostling over well-worn stones while the sun slowly warms our back and a chorus of birds lulls us to sleep. Of course there are things to avoid, but maybe a bit more environmental exposure is just what the doctor needs to order. We will discuss some of the basic principles to help manage your environmental exposure in chapter 12.

Habits and Hygiene:

This sphere of Lifestyle Synergy is pretty straightforward and obvious but extremely important for both acute and chronic disease prevention. Proper hygiene habits are a hallmark of disease prevention, but as most of our mothers taught us as we grew up, they will only help us if we actually practice them regularly. Keeping ourselves and our surroundings clean, washing our hands after using the bathroom, and practicing oral hygiene are the basics, but we should also avoid habits and behaviors known to increase risk, such as smoking, illicit drug use, and promiscuity. We won't try to nag, but we will give you some basic principles in chapter 13.

Community and Purpose:

A huge part of just being human (and a healthy human at that) comes through the larger interactions with those around us. How we structure our life and our relationships has an amazing influence on many of the other spheres of Lifestyle Synergy. Eating a meal with a tightly knit, loving family has much more impact on a toddler than merely the macronutrient content on the plate. Staying up late worrying about how to manage a stressful job during a messy divorce and child custody dispute will overwhelm the many great signals coming from a well-balanced salad. When it comes to our health, no man (or woman) is an island.

Ultimately, our health is a means to an end, not an end in itself. Those without purpose, a deeper understanding of why they exist, will either ruin themselves and their health or, conversely, view their own health as a trophy for the mantel. Every day that our health keeps us well enough to pursue that great purpose for which we are designed, we are blessed. When our energy, time, and money are consumed in keeping us from debility or worse, just holding death at bay for a few more years, it is difficult to pursue our true God-given purpose, and we and others suffer the consequences. There are few things more damaging to our health than hopelessness and lack of purpose; when we lose the will to live, we don't stop to read the nutrition labels on our food or the warning labels on our cartons of cigarettes. In chapter 14, we will explore basic principles that will help put health into perspective and help guide you to a greater purpose.

The Prevention-to-Intervention Hierarchy

If this book were written simply as a way to discuss lifestyle as a means to *prevent* disease alone, this section wouldn't be necessary. I can't imagine, however, that this book will often find its way into the hands of someone under twenty years old with no health worries. To paraphrase an old adage—good health is wasted on the young. Most of the time, people don't start thinking about prevention until they notice changes in their own health or the health of someone close to them. In our river analogy from chapter 5, they don't begin to paddle until they have allowed the subtle currents of life to cause their canoe to drift a bit downstream. At that point they need both prevention and intervention. Thankfully, the same lifestyle decisions that maintain our health can, with a modest increase in dose and intensity, become powerful tools for intervention. In fact, regardless of how much our health has deteriorated, lifestyle solutions should always be at the core of our prevention and intervention strategies. We will explain further as we describe the Prevention-to-Intervention Hierarchy.

Lifestyle Maintenance

If we imagine our health surrounded by a protective fence supported by our seven spheres of Lifestyle Synergy, you have a picture of what I call lifestyle maintenance. The signals coming from each of these spheres create the dynamic balance that we call health and do so without our conscious effort. Health, unlike *dis-ease*, mostly goes unnoticed.

Maintaining a healthy system, just like paddling in the wide part of the river, seems effortless. When our metabolic reserves are at high capacity and our physiological resilience is strong, our health is easily maintained by prudent living. At this stage in our prevention-to-intervention hierarchy, we rely upon the power of repetitive, low-dose signaling coming from each of the seven spheres. We don't need radical diets or exercise programs at this stage to maintain the system. In fact, moderation and balance are what we need.

To be sure, the power of lifestyle maintenance is affected, in part, by our genes (including epigenic influences) and uncontrollable environmental influences. Along with our daily lifestyle decisions, these factors influence the pressure placed upon our physiological resilience—the buffering capacity every system relies upon to keep our health comfortably "inside the fence." If we consistently fail to make good lifestyle decisions, we decrease the good signals and increase the harmful signals to our cells and tissues. We simply succumb to the current of the river when we stop paddling the canoe. If we notice that we have drifted, we can now pick up the paddle and begin moving back upstream. At this stage, our lifestyle decisions are meant not only to maintain our position but as a means to prevent us from moving any farther downstream. We call this lifestyle intervention.

Lifestyle Intervention

When the medical community thinks about lifestyle medicine, what they usually mean is lifestyle intervention, which implies that some form of lifestyle change will be used to intervene to prevent a condition from getting worse or to reduce the risk for some disease in the future (like diabetes in the Diabetes Prevention Program). In fact, lifestyle intervention studies are usually categorized as either *moderate* or *intense* based on the "dose" of the lifestyle change being implemented. It is important to understand, for the paradigm being laid out in this book, that the mechanisms driving lifestyle intervention are the same as the mechanisms driving lifestyle maintenance. The basic difference is the intensity and the intentionality of the lifestyle choices being made.

When we begin to assess the "fence" that keeps our health from wandering astray, we may notice a breach, an area left neglected and in need of repair. Perhaps a decade (or two) passes by without much intentional physical activity. Add to that poor sleeping habits and a bit of stress, and we have described the lifestyle of the average 40-year-old American. Some may be worse off than others, depending both upon their specific genetic make-up and on how much metabolic reserve they amassed before drifting downstream. All of a sudden, what starts out as a fairly routine medical check-up, perhaps for an overdue life insurance policy, turns into a series of critical questions for both patient and clinician.

Now what? As patients continue to drift farther from what they weighed at their high school graduation, the lab reports start showing some disturbing trends. Blood glucose and lipids are up, and so is the marker that measures inflammation (C-reactive protein). Blood pressure is on the incline, while energy is on the decline. This scene plays out thousands of times per day across the clinics of our land, as 70 million Americans have pre-hypertension and over 100 million people have metabolic syndrome—a precursor to both diabetes and cardiovascular disease. Many of these individuals will walk out of their doctors' offices with a prescription. What will be written on that piece of paper? Will it be a description of a diet and physical activity program designed to reduce their specific risk profile? Will it be a recommendation on how to improve their sleep and reduce the amount of stress affecting their health? If statistics hold true, it is unlikely to have any of these recommendations; instead it will need to be deciphered by a pharmacist before being filled.

As we will outline in the chapters ahead, concerted (and synergistic) lifestyle intervention programs are far and away the most powerful tools to prevent and reverse most chronic disease processes, even after they have progressed enough to change lab values. And even if a clinician or patient determines that other therapies should be added (i.e. nutritional supplementation, chiropractic care, pharmaceuticals), a foundational therapy involving lifestyle intervention continues to be the basis for improving physiological resilience and recharging metabolic reserve.

For that 40-year-old we mentioned earlier, whose health was diminished because of the absence of signals coming from physical activity, proper sleep, and stress management, this might mean a specific effort to get off the couch and to begin increasing the signals that come from good physical activity, sleep, and appropriate management of stress. As we increase the signals coming from the neglected spheres of lifestyle synergy, bringing them once again into balance with all the others, healthy outcomes are inevitable.

Augmenting Lifestyle: A Targeted Approach

Change is difficult. Interventions that rely on changing personal behavior are always fraught with the issue of "compliance." In fact, one of the reasons many clinicians give lifestyle therapies the cold shoulder might be boiled down to something like, "Sure, it might work, but my patients won't/can't sustain those kinds of changes for very long." Perhaps; but what sort of tools and motivation usually accompany the advice to change lifestyle behavior? Studies suggest it is very little. On the other hand, we need to take seriously this fundamental difficulty that humans have in changing their ways. Add to this the fact that many individuals are already suffering from the consequences of neglected chronic diseases when they make their first appointment. They want to see tangible results in a timely manner.

Here I advocate for what I call augmented lifestyle intervention. While lifestyle intervention is still at the heart, we often need to augment this approach with therapies that are specific and targeted to complement the mechanisms at the core of lifestyle medicine. Augmented lifestyle intervention, when appropriately applied, can speed up the progress toward health and act as a potent prevention against deteriorating chronic disease. This approach includes a host of intervention strategies such as nutritional supplementation, nutraceutical therapies, chiropractic and related therapies, certain detoxification protocols, physical therapy, and a host of other techniques and modalities. I have spent the last sixteen years supporting clinicians who practice these types of interventions and have been amazed to see how powerful they can be.

When we understand just how the body turns the many signals from lifestyle into health, it is possible to find specific signals driving the health outcome that are more potent than others. For example, the nutrigenomic example we mentioned previously showed that the flavonoid quercetin is one of the key signaling molecules we get from eating certain plants. While we can rely on our diet to provide high levels of quercetin and related compounds (and we should), we can also augment our diet by providing higher doses of quercetin in the form of capsules, tablets, or powders. In fact, in high doses, quercetin acts as a powerful mast-cell stabilizing agent, which can help reduce how sensitive we are to airborne and other allergens.[†] While it might be possible to get this same anti-allergy effect by consuming foods containing high levels of quercetin (like yellow onions), by augmenting our diet with this flavonoid in capsule form we might get results that are significantly faster and more powerful.

There are literally thousands of examples we could give in addition to quercetin to describe the benefits of this approach. We will only

---

[†] So powerful are the mast-cell stabilizing effects of flavonoids like quercetin that a synthetic flavonoid-analog, sodium cromelyn, was created by the pharmaceutical industry years ago to mimic this effect. In head-to-head cell culture studies, however, quercetin outperforms its synthetic cousin, which also has the unenviable property of being virtually un-absorbable.

Figure 7.2 **The Prevention-Intervention Hierachy**

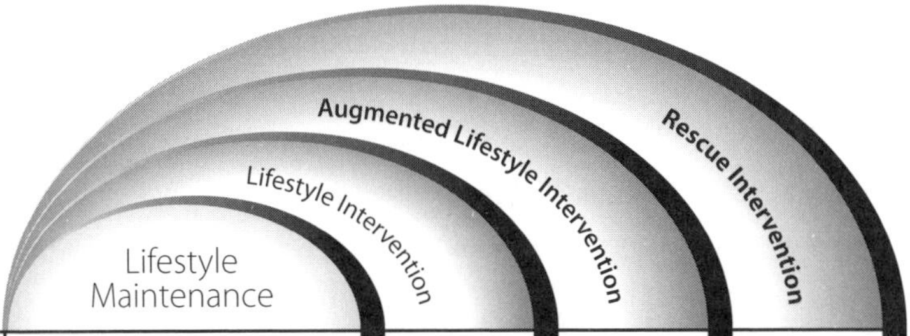

	Lifestyle Maintenance	Lifestyle Intervention	Augmented Lifestyle Intervention	Rescue Intervention
Vitamin D & Bones	Sunlight: Work and Play	Sun Therapy/ Diet	Vitamin D Supplement	Osteoporosis Drugs
Antioxidant Defense	Wholesome Diverse Diet	↑ Fruits & Veggies	Supplement Lipoic Acid/ Quercetin etc.	?
Back Health	Normal Physical Activity	Exercise and Flex Training	Chiropractic/ Physical Therapy	Surgery/Pain Medications
Joint Health	Physical Activity/Hydration	Weight Loss/ Flexibility	Glucosamine/ Chondroitin Sulfate	Drugs, Knee Replacement
Cancer Prevention	Wholesome Diverse Diet	↑ Fruits & Veggies (Cruciferous)	Supplement Sulforophane or I3C	Antineoplastic Drugs
Detoxification	Wholesome Living	Avoidance/ Organic Focus	Supplement Agents that ↑Detoxification	Drugs to Combat Toxin Symptoms

These are just a few examples of how the various levels of intervention are rooted in Lifestyle-based intervention and signaling.

describe some of these, giving examples for each sphere of our model throughout the next seven chapters; Figure 7.2 shows some general examples to give an overall picture of how this principle works.

For the vast number of Americans over 40 (and a good portion of those who are younger), augmented lifestyle intervention is the only way to reach their goals of prevention and intervention in a timely fashion, in many cases helping them to limit or avoid the need for rescue interventions (described next) to prevent irreversible end-organ damage or death.

Rescue Intervention

While the most powerful tool to maintain our health is provided by signals that work with our body's innate healing capacity, the majority of dollars in the healthcare and medical research systems are spent in the discovery and use of agents that attempt to impose a solution upon health problems. This is rescue intervention. Think of it like a net placed at the edge of a waterfall that prevents the canoe from crashing to the bottom. Rescue intervention can certainly play a role in chronic disease management by delaying end-organ damage and death.[†] While this can be a valuable tool in the alleviation of suffering, this should not be confused with making someone fundamentally *healthier*.

Consider just some of the rescue interventions in cardiology alone: stents, coronary artery by-pass grafts, implantable defibrillators and ventricular valve replacement, even transplants. It is pretty amazing how far our technologies have come, yet rarely is someone fundamentally *healthier* as a result of getting such intervention. Often these interventions are the only viable options keeping someone from major debilitation or death; and for that we are grateful to have them available. The problem arises when, enamored with their role as a rescue intervention, we attempt to apply them as if they could actually prevent or even reverse chronic disease. To use our analogy once again, it would be like thinking the net that prevents the canoe from going over the waterfall can actually help paddle the canoe back upstream. More often than not, additional medications must be given to these patients to ameliorate the effects (side effects) of the rescue intervention itself. In our intervention hierarchy, the closer we are to the core of lifestyle maintenance, the fewer side effects we experience.

Since rescue interventions such as pharmaceuticals, surgery, and medical devices rarely increase metabolic reserve (often depleting it) or improve physiological resilience, the goal of the Lifestyle Synergy approach is to rely mainly upon core lifestyle-driven solutions—the signals our bodies are designed to receive and interpret, augmented with appropriate therapies as needed.

---

† Our intervention hierarchy is intended to describe *chronic* disease prevention and intervention. Emergency medicine, with its vast array of technological advances, is a valuable form of rescue intervention we would not want to live without.

The Principles of Lifestyle Synergy

There is no end to the books that have been written to tell you exactly what to eat, how to lose weight, and a myriad of other behavioral activities. The goal of this project is not to dictate every minute detail of your life, but instead to prescribe principles upon which you can design a healthy life. These principles are designed to help you focus on activities that improve the number of good lifestyle signals while diminishing the number of bad lifestyle signals so your body can accomplish the rest.

Principle #1: You can't obtain good health by overdoing one sphere of intervention while neglecting the others. The sum is greater than the parts. This is the advantage of synergy.

If I asked a farmer to name the single most important ingredient for an abundant and healthy crop, would he choose the seed or the soil? How about sunlight, rain, nutrient density, absence of pests, or the timing of the harvest? Any one of these things could sink the crop, but none of them can completely overcome the failures of the others. If he spent all his money purchasing the best seed in the world but planted it in the poorest soil, the outcome might actually be worse than had he purchased lesser quality seeds and planted them in good soil. This reminds me of the days when young athletes would spend so much time working on their physique and training, virtually ignoring their dietary habits. Even though they were young and had great metabolic reserve, they realized that neglecting their diet would soon diminish the gains they were making in the gym. Emphasizing one area of health to the neglect of others is a bad long-term strategy.

A great illustration of the phenomenon of Lifestyle Synergy was published in 2011 amongst the many finding of the Nurse's Health Study. One of the largest studies on a cohort of women, followed now for over 30 years, the Nurse's Health Study has tracked the health and lifestyle habits of over 81,000 female nurses in the U.S. While hundreds of papers have been published from data derived from this study (we mentioned one in chapter 4 about nut consumption and diabetes), the following example is one of the most profound in respect to the power of the synergy of lifestyle intervention.[3]

As it turns out, sudden cardiac death (SCD) accounts for more than half of all cardiac deaths in women, with an incidence of approximately 250,000 to 310,000 cases annually in the United States. If we are looking for a definitive end-point to measure, this would be it. What these researchers did was correlate a few easily measured lifestyle factors with the incidence of SCD in these nurses between 1984 and 2010. In fact, while SCD is linked to many potential lifestyle factors, the researchers chose just four: smoking habits, body mass index (BMI), diet score, and the amount of regular physical activity. In each of these 4 lifestyle factors, a relative score was given for high- or low-risk behavior. The *lowest* risk for each factor respectively was never smoking, BMI less than 25, diet in the top 40% of a Mediterranean diet score, and at least thirty minutes of moderate to vigorous physical activity per day.

Now here is where the synergy part works. For those nurses who were in the lowest risk group for just one of these four factors, their probability of sudden cardiac death was reduced by 40% relative to the women who were unable to meet any of the low-risk behaviors. This sounds pretty impressive until you realize that the women who maintained a low-risk lifestyle in all four categories had a whopping 92% decrease in their risk for SCD. There is no drug that could come close to achieving this kind of preventative potential. In fact, the statisticians who looked at this data said that if these four factors were considered the direct cause of the deaths in these women, they calculated that SCD in women is over 80% preventable by lifestyle behaviors alone. Let us be clear; even though these researchers only measured four aspects of prudent lifestyle behavior, you can imagine how many other lifestyle behaviors were likely to have been associated with these factors.

As you read through the rest of these chapters, you might realize that your personal health focus has been isolated to only a few of the seven spheres of lifestyle intervention. It is not uncommon for someone to focus on one, perhaps diet, to the exclusion of the others, not realizing that they act in a synergistic way. As you come across principles that seem a bit more difficult or challenging, think about how to incorporate even modest changes in those areas to synergize with the others you may already have down pat.

Principle #2: When it comes to prevention, the earlier the better; but it's never too late to leverage lifestyle intervention.

If you are an ambitious teenager reading these pages, congratulations—you have more foresight than the average American. Regrettably, most people don't really start thinking about their health until it begins to wane, which used to be at about forty years old. As we discussed previously, the onset of metabolic diseases like insulin resistance, obesity, diabetes, and heart disease is occurring in younger and younger populations with each passing decade. The metabolic reserve doesn't seem to last as long as it once did. We explained why this is in chapter 5. Recall that the synergy of poor lifestyle habits is at an all-time high and, when coupled with the accumulation of heritable epigenic influences, has made each generation more susceptible to these chronic metabolic disorders.

Early lifestyle intervention strategies can not only prevent chronic disease in those individuals willing to implement them, but by starting early enough, the negative epigenetic influence upon their genes can actually be altered, reducing the next generation's risk for the same outcomes. In both generations, the earlier the preventative steps begin, the more powerful the outcome. If you are a parent reading this book and you want healthy grandchildren, start talking with your pre-teens about ways to maintain their health or about reversing any unhealthy patterns that have already become part of their life. The power of prevention should be maximized in the young, whose metabolic reserve is highest.

That is well and good if you're young, but what about those of us over 40? Fortunately, there is some great news here. The most powerful tool to maintain our health (or reverse our drift) is still lifestyle intervention; it just requires a bit more focus and attention than when we were younger (it's always harder paddling up the stream). Remember the Diabetes Prevention Program (DPP) study we discussed earlier, which showed that lifestyle intervention was twice as effective in reducing the risk for diabetes over four years compared to the drug metformin in pre-diabetic subjects?[4] Well, as it turns out, if you look at the DPP subjects, you might be a bit surprised by the influence of age on the treatment outcome. In each of the "younger" age groups (25–44 years old and 45–59 years old) researchers found that lifestyle intervention exceeded the benefit of the drug metformin, although both were able to reduce the incidence of diabetes. On the other hand, with the subjects over 60 years of age, metformin had no effect whatsoever on the incidence of diabetes (no statistical difference from the group given the placebo), while lifestyle intervention was actually more potent in reducing diabetes incidence in this age group.

Figure 7.3 **The Effect of Age on DPP Outcomes**

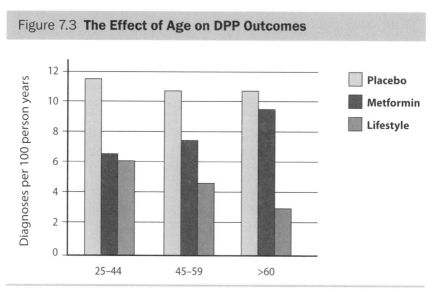

Note that while both metformin and lifestyle are equally powerful to reduce risk in the younger patients, lifestyle therapy continues to become more powerful in each of the older age groups while metformin ceases to be effective in patients over 60.

It turns out that when you look into the details of the results of the DPP, the older subjects were more compliant for every recommendation. They lost more weight, kept the weight off longer, exercised more, and attended more motivational meetings than any of the other age groups. What the elderly might lack in metabolic reserve they can overcome with diligence and compliance; and their cells are still ready to respond. So while you may have neglected your health for decades, don't think that rescue interventions are your only hope to prevent or reverse serious chronic illness. It may require a concerted effort of lifestyle changes along with targeted augmentation therapies, but if you have read this far into this book, you are likely serious enough about your health to make substantial alterations.

Principle #3: A healthy lifestyle pattern reduces ALL chronic disease risk. The side effect of Lifestyle Synergy is more health.

As you will see throughout each of the next chapters, it is downright uncanny how research has shown that a similar pattern of prudent lifestyle decisions reduces the risk of a broad range of chronic diseases. Unlike the rescue interventions that are extremely specific in their effect and usage (drugs are only approved for use in patients with specific conditions), lifestyle interventions have an almost universal benefit. For instance, a diet that improves lipid levels and reduces inflammatory markers will result in the reduction of cardiovascular disease, diabetes, Alzheimer's disease, and cancer, just to name a few of the most studied chronic diseases. If we implement lifestyle as a pattern of good decisions, the balance of (mostly) good signals will offset the limited number of bad signals sent to our cells. Of course, after seeing how chronic diseases develop and how the signals produced by lifestyle inputs tell our cells to function, this "panacea" effect of lifestyle should come as no surprise.

The one misconception many clinicians and patients accept is thinking that there are completely different lifestyle interventions for each disease condition. This idea, spurred on by the vast number of books and recommendations published each year that appear to suggest different protocols for each disease, can lead to confusion and futility. The notion that vastly different lifestyle intervention approaches would be required to prevent each different chronic disease is contrary to both reason and the scientific literature. Is there room for nuance? Of course there is, but we don't want to miss the forest for the trees.

When we talk about a pattern, we don't mean that every lifestyle decision will affect every individual in the exact same way. We are talking about principles, not dogmatic absolutes. Remember that our systems are resilient and can compensate for a range of responses. Even if one person has an allergy to a particular food, requiring them to avoid its consumption, the next person might find it an important part of their daily diet. What one person finds stress-reducing, another might find very stressful. While a particular exercise may be considered strenuous and therefore beneficial for one person, another person might get very little benefit from it. When you understand and implement the basic patterns driving good health first, there is ample enough time to experiment with nuances that can help augment the success of lifestyle intervention in each person.

Principle #4: Give lifestyle intervention enough time to work—you didn't get here overnight.

This principle seems straightforward enough but often frustrates those clinicians and patients waiting for the "results." After twenty years or more of stretching our physiological resilience with poor lifestyle habits, why are we surprised when it doesn't just snap back after a few months of prudence? The capacity for health is still there; we just need to maintain those good signals, steady and consistent, to begin the rebuilding process. Most of the time you can speed things up by using augmented lifestyle intervention therapies, but the longer someone's health has been neglected, the longer it will likely take to reach their goals.

Unfortunately, our research models just aren't designed to wait very long for the results. Because research is often so expensive, many clinical trials attempt to reach statistically significant results in as little as a few weeks or months. This short timeframe might suit some of the mechanisms displayed by powerful rescue interventions, which might be capable of altering disease-specific biomarkers within hours, days, or weeks—long before their side effects typically manifest. On the other hand, studies that last long enough to demonstrate the benefits of lifestyle intervention show that those benefits last even when the therapy is stopped.

Again, the DPP trial is a great example. While the intervention officially lasted four years, the groups were followed for a total of ten years.[5] Even though the weight lost in the first year of the intervention was mostly regained in the subsequent nine years, and all three groups ended the ten years with similar weight loss, those initially in the lifestyle arm of the study had a significantly lower incidence of diabetes than either the placebo or metformin arm at the end of the ten-year period (six years after the trial was over). This extended benefit, which has been described in other studies, has been dubbed the "legacy effect" by many of the researchers in the field. What this phenomenon suggests is that a recharging of the metabolic reserve occurs when we implement intensive lifestyle intervention. This is rarely true of rescue interventions, which cease to be effective when they are stopped or actually cause a strong rebound of the metabolite or biomarker they were intended to manage.

Always remember that lifestyle is a prescription for life and for a lifetime—there will be times of more intense compliance and times when it will seem you are pulled downstream by the current. Don't give up just because you don't see the expected results right away—you are likely making more progress than you think.

Principle #5: Everything in moderation, even lifestyle intervention. You can get too much of a good thing.

Just because something provides good signals to the cells, it doesn't mean that the cells can't be overwhelmed by those signals. As we will see when we look at the seven spheres in detail, moderation and balance are the keys to using lifestyle as an intervention tool. In fact, many signals trigger a series of feedback mechanisms that actually limit their own effects; sometimes high doses can actually be harmful. At the very least, there is a diminishing return for most good signals.

In some cases, this principle is obvious. Choosing the best foods but consuming them in excess will limit their overall benefit. Getting enough sunlight to give us optimized levels of vitamin D is one thing, but excessive sunlight can obviously damage our skin. And so it is with sleep duration, exercise intensity, vitamin supplementation, socialization, and a myriad of lifestyle decisions—there is usually a point when more is no longer helpful or perhaps even harmful to our health.

This dynamic can be described in what is often called the "U-shaped curve" (Figure 7.4). Most beneficial signals have some sort of dose response that continues to increase as the dose of that substance increases. In fact, most experiments, whether they are done in test tubes, in animals, or in humans, aim to show that the substance they are researching is responsible for the benefit they are describing. One obvious way to suggest causation is to show a dose-response effect related to the substance. If the effect being measured is not changed when the dose of the substance is changed, many would question if benefit was linked to the substance at all.

Figure 7.4 **Different Dose-Response Curves**

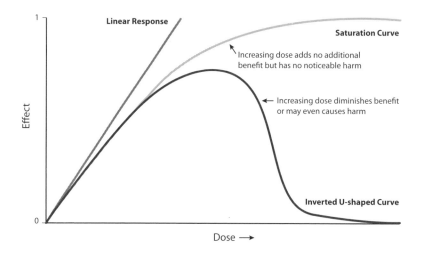

There are three basic dynamics that occur as dose increases. Rarely is there a linear relationship, where improvement continues as higher and higher doses are given. For most everything, there is either a saturation curve or an inverse "U-shaped" curve. Both show that at some point, increasing doses cease to increase the beneficial effect; however, as the inverted U-shape curves shows, increased doses of many things will actually diminish benefit or even cause harm.

What we often find in those studies is that there is a defined range at which the benefit continues to increase as the dose increases. Then, either gradually or abruptly, that benefit stops increasing or actually diminishes. This principle is important to understand for a number of reasons. The first we have already mentioned: that good signals can be overdone and might even turn into bad signals as they overload the system they are intended to benefit. Another is the fact that the dose range for effective responses might be higher or lower depending on the patient or their situation. As you begin to put these lifestyle principles to work, try different "doses" of change to see how you respond. Listen to your body; it will often tell you when you are overdoing something. It doesn't mean you need to stop altogether; you just may need to reduce the dose for a while.

Principle #6: Find a companion for your journey; life is meant to be shared. With lifestyle medicine, there is strength in numbers.

There are few places I would rather avoid than the average waiting room in the average clinic: a dozen or so people who have never met, sitting around awkwardly, avoiding each other's glances, waiting for their names to be announced before being marched back to exam room number 3 on the left. Alone now, each one anxiously awaits the clinician while sitting uncomfortably and awkwardly on the roll of paper covering the exam table. This is the interface with medicine that most people experience: institutional and isolated.

Let's face it, the setting in which most of medicine takes place is simply not warm and fuzzy. In such a setting, it is difficult to have a good "bedside manner," even for clinicians with the best of intentions. Some clinics understand this and are beginning to change; most people, however, still experience what is described above.

The balance between privacy on the one hand and isolation on the other is a challenge in today's medical model. Lifestyle medicine, like life itself, is meant to be shared. So it should come as no surprise that some of the most successful lifestyle intervention models come from studies using group therapy rather than individual care alone. The camaraderie, both from the encouragement received and from the ability to encourage others, creates an environment of healing. The advantages of group sessions are not only for the patient; the clinic can gain many benefits as well, not the least of which is greater success with its patients.

Imagine you are a clinician and you really want to spend the time telling all your patients about the wonderful things you know about diet and exercise, sleep, and stress management to help them lose weight and stop their drift toward diabetes. With the five to ten minutes you get with the patient, you only have enough time to review the records, ask about current complaints, and complete your physical examination before moving to the next room. Perhaps you show them a pamphlet or quickly tell them about a recent book you like, but you wish you had more time.

What many clinics are discovering is that many of these patients will gladly return for a scheduled group session tailored to their particular condition. Now at one time and for all to hear, a clinician or staff member can discuss all the details they want about diet, exercise, stress management, and sleep.[†] Not only does this allow the clinician to give a substantial amount of time to these subjects, they can do so in a very efficient manner. Patients often thrive in this atmosphere because they can ask questions, share anecdotes, and find others who struggle with similar conditions. As in most other areas of our lives, we tend to gravitate toward others who can understand and support us. Why should our health be any different?

If you are reading this book and attempting to implement major life changes from the principles learned within, look around your life and ask yourself: "Who can I take along as a companion on this journey?" They might not need to make all the same changes you are attempting, but they can encourage you in the process and likely have some others to work on themselves.

[†] Usually an informed consent form is filled out by all participants so that each person present agrees to hold confidential any medical information shared by another participant in the group.

CHAPTER 8

Let Food Be Your Medicine: Diet as Intervention

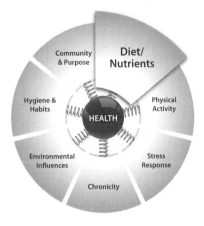

"No disease that can be treated by diet should be treated with any other means."

—Maimonides (1135–1204)

IF YOU HAVE HAD the opportunity to travel to out-of-the way parts of the planet, you know that few things define a culture like its food. Villages just a few miles from each other may have very different cuisines and cooking styles, many of which help distinguish them from their close neighbors. Certain foods can be sacred, used in special ceremonies or religious rites, and nearly every culture celebrates with feasting, fasting, or both. In the West, and especially in the United States, we have access to a wide variety of cultural foods, although many of these have been modified to our portion sizes and tastes. With all these options, we still have preferences that define our eating patterns—our favorite foods. I am always reminded of this fact when my children attempt to get to know someone. Invariably, after their name and favorite color, they always seem to ask about their favorite food, almost as if, instinctively, they understand that the answer to this question speaks to the core of someone's personality.

So our diet is not only part of what defines us culturally; for many it is intensely personal. If you are not convinced that someone's food preferences are a critical part of their life, ask them to change their diet and find out what happens. As one person told me, "Friends don't tell friends what foods to eat." We bristle at the concept that we might be contributing to our own future disease risk just by eating the foods "we have always eaten." Could there be something about our eating habits (and appetites) that is rooted in our will?

I've always found it intriguing that the biblical account of the first human sin revolved around "eating" of the forbidden fruit. Amongst the first instructions recorded in Genesis was a clear dietary restriction! "*Thou shalt not eat…*" was the command, but they ate anyway.† While there are numerous theological implications behind these events in the Garden of Eden, I don't believe it to be coincidental that this particular restriction proved difficult for humankind. Later, the scriptures record the definition of specific "clean" and "unclean" foods that would help maintain the chosen people as a "separate" and holy nation apart from the nations around them. Their diet, among other distinctions, would define them.

The cruel irony is that even when we have convinced ourselves that we need to change what we are eating, we find our dietary patterns are often harder to adjust than we thought. When we start a new diet, we often focus our attentions on the "forbidden fruits" rather than on the myriad foods that are permitted. Like Adam and Eve, we define ourselves by what we can't have (I am on a gluten-free, dairy-free, fat-free, low-carb diet, etc.). Think about it: the average American will consume in the neighborhood of fifty to eighty tons of food in their lifetime. If we

---

† The "fall" of Adam and Eve, one of the most well-known stories in history, is described in Genesis 2 and 3. The fruit, often depicted as an apple, is never described except to say that the tree it came from was "*a delight to the eyes.*" How well the marketers of foods today know that the first organ of the appetite is the eye.

could convert this amount of food into the number of signals provided to our cells, it would be an astronomically large number. Like tiny drops of water on a massive rock, each signal seems to have no perceptible effect, but together they can carve a trough even in the hardest granite.

This chapter will focus on the key principles that allow you to create healthy foundations for your dietary and nutritional decisions. You have plenty of decisions to make—in fact several tons (literally) of food decisions in your future. These principles should help you make the best of those decisions.

Principle #1: Choose a healthy dietary pattern that governs 80% of your decisions. The Mediterranean pattern is one of the best and most diverse.

This first principle is absolutely foundational if you are to sustain your health into the future with nutrition, so we will spend a little more time unpacking the details. When it comes to diet and nutrition, it is about *the pattern* of food choices that guide your eating decisions—*the majority of the time.* You should not be "on a diet" but instead following a dietary pattern. You need to consciously select a healthy eating pattern and arrange your dietary decisions so that you can maintain this pattern for 80% of your meals and snacks.†

This might mean that 80% of *each meal* conforms to your healthy pattern, or perhaps 80% of your meals each week, so if we assume that you eat three meals per day, this would mean that seventeen of those twenty-one meals would be described as part of this pattern. It also means (I am sure some have already done the math) that four meals per week would not necessarily need to follow this pattern. A few excursions off the pristine path (even planned excursions) are unlikely to ruin the benefit of the 80%, as long as you don't use these four meals to binge on foods that derail the benefit of the other seventeen.

This principle also means that most of the foods in your cupboards, refrigerator, freezer, and grocery cart should be consistent with this

---

† We chose 80% based on Pareto's principle, the "80/20 rule," often used to determine impact in an organizational setting. For a business, this principle describes the need to understand what decisions and customers impact 80% of their business—often it is 20% of their clients. Churches will also tell you that 80% of the volunteer help often comes from the same 20% of the congregants.

healthy eating pattern. As we will see later, having an abundance of foods readily available that are outside of your healthy pattern can often overwhelm even the best of intentions.

Without thinking, most of us choose to eat the foods we grew up with because they are familiar, they comfort us, and we know how to prepare them. I think most Americans would find it difficult to describe the dietary pattern they follow even though it may be leading to their demise. I challenge you to keep a food diary, writing down everything you eat and drink for a whole week. Or look at a month's worth of grocery bills and highlight those items that are healthy and those that are unhealthy. Whether you like it or not, this is your current dietary pattern. You have the power to choose what you eat most of the time—what is it going to be?

Traits of a Healthy and Successful Dietary Pattern

- Improves all health outcomes
- Is easy to implement with available foods
- Works with the body's natural healing capacity
- Includes a diversity of colors and textures
- Tastes great and satisfies hunger
- Can be maintained on almost any budget

Why the Mediterranean diet?

For centuries, physicians, scientists, and laypeople have been in pursuit of the optimal diet, one that promotes healthy aging and prevents all chronic disease. While many dietary patterns have shown themselves to be superior in one way or another, the one pattern most extensively researched in Western populations, with data to support its efficacy in preventing almost every major chronic disease, is the Mediterranean diet (MedDiet).[†] In contrast with typical Western diets, which have been repeatedly associated with an increased risk for nearly every chronic disease, epidemiological studies have found that the Mediterranean dietary pattern is significantly protective against a wide range of

---

† Other dietary patterns have also been studied, some with better outcomes than others. They include the standard American diet (SAD), vegetarian/vegan, low-fat, low-carbohydrate, the so-called Paleolithic diet, the macrobiotic diet, and a host of other diets described in popular books or as guideline recommendations by groups such as the American Heart Association.

chronic diseases such as heart disease, diabetes, obesity, neurological and cognitive decline, and even cancer.[1,2] Increasingly, studies are also showing that this dietary pattern is a legitimate intervention strategy in populations across the globe, lending key support to the importance of diet/lifestyle in the prevention and treatment of chronic disease.

So what is a MedDiet? Essentially, it describes the basic eating patterns of the peoples living around the Mediterranean Sea, a very diverse population of ethnicities, cultures, and culinary backgrounds. This broad definition has become more specific as researchers attempt to describe healthy eating patterns. The first modern study to define the health benefits of the MedDiet was the Seven Countries Study, a large thirty-year study that included 13,000 subjects in sixteen different study groups from around the world. Amongst all the different groups from around the globe, the Crete cohort emerged as the population with the lowest rate of heart disease, and among the many features driving this reduced risk for cardiovascular illness were the lifestyle and dietary patterns of this population.[3–5]

For decades, the benefits of the MedDiet were known exclusively to the epidemiologists and researchers doing this type of research and a handful of clinicians familiar with these early studies.[3,4] It was not until Harvard researcher Walter Willett published his popular book *Eat, Drink and Be Healthy* that the MedDiet became part of the broader dietary discussion here in the United States.[6] Willett and his colleagues consistently found that diets comprised of saturated fat, trans-fatty acids, high glycemic load, and low intake of vegetables (measured as low-folate consumption) were associated with an increased risk of coronary heart disease (CHD), while diets consisting of higher amounts of polyunsaturated fatty acids (PUFA) and monounsaturated fatty acids (MUFA), omega-3 fatty acids, and higher intakes of fruits and vegetables were associated with lower CHD risk.[7,8]

The traditional Greek MedDiet is low in saturated fats and high in monounsaturated fat (primarily from the omega-9 oleic acid from olive oil), with a ratio of unsaturated:saturated fat of around 2 or more. This is not a low-fat dietary pattern. In fact, total fat in the MedDiet may reach 40% of total energy intake, mostly from olive oil. Neither is the diet low in carbohydrates, but the carbs are usually low in their glycemic impact since they are derived from complex carbohydrates such as whole grains and legumes and fiber (mainly from vegetables and fruits). The diet also includes dairy, mostly cheese and yogurt, and ample fish consumption due to the region's proximity to the sea.[9] This diverse dietary pattern provides a high intake of carotenoids, B-vitamins, tocopherols (vitamin E family), minerals, and a number of diverse healthy plant compounds called phytonutrients (like the flavonoid quercetin). It should be noted that, for the most part, the traditional MedDiet is absent of refined and packaged foods.

Epidemiological evidence concurs; increased adherence to this diverse traditional diet has been repeatedly associated with a reduced risk of overall and cardiovascular mortality, reduced cancer incidence and mortality, and lower incidence of Parkinson's and Alzheimer's diseases.[10] Higher adherence to the MedDiet has been so effective that there is now a MedDiet score researchers use to measure a healthy dietary pattern in clinical research.[11] The high phytonutrient content and substitution of refined and high glycemic-impact foods with monounsaturated fats and healthy carbohydrates and proteins are largely responsible for the positive data on lower heart disease and diabetes risk factors in those following a MedDiet. The diet has been also shown to help modulate immune cell activation and decrease concentrations of inflammatory biomarkers such as C-reactive protein, both important factors in avoiding cardiometabolic risk.[12]

While it is true that researchers have been exploring how each dietary component of the MedDiet (i.e. olive oil, nuts, fish, fruit, vegetables, spices, etc.) influences human health, none has been able to replicate the benefit of the diet as a whole. A healthy and diverse dietary pattern is, by definition, a synergistic approach virtually impossible to break apart into its component signals. As we saw earlier, the science of nutrigenomics can tell us how each dietary component creates a part of the whole response (up-regulating or down-regulating genes, etc.), even helping us choose some of these components for augmented nutritional and nutraceutical therapies. In the end, however, each of these components is limited when attempting to provide the benefits of the whole pattern. The sum is always greater than the parts.

Tips for Decreasing Glycemic Impact

When implementing a MedDiet, low glycemic-impact carbohydrates should comprise 40–50% of calories, protein should comprise another 20–30%, and fats 30%. Patients with type 2 diabetes or insulin resistance should consider an even lower glycemic impact version of the MedDiet, staying close to 40% carbohydrates (concentrating on only low glycemic-index carbohydrates), 30% protein, and 30% fats.

- Reduce the frequency of refined carbohydrate consumption (i.e. white bread, white pasta, muffins, cakes, and cookies) and focus instead on whole grain-based foods (such as bulgur, rice, quinoa, and wheat berries) as well as legumes/plant proteins (such as beans and lentils) and whole grains.
- Increase soluble and fermentable fiber content through your diet or through supplementation. Fermentable fibers are things like inulin and fructoligosaccharides (FOS).
- Increase phytonutrients by using brightly colored vegetables, fruits, spices, and herbs and moderate intake of juice from fruits with high polyphenol content such as grapes, berries, or pomegranates.
- Use spices to improve insulin sensitivity as well as monounsaturated fats in the form of nuts, olive oil, and avocados.
- Do not skip breakfast, as this meal sets the metabolic foundation for the rest of the day (this is so important it is principle #3 below).
- Consider small, high-protein snacks between meals to keep blood sugar stable.
- Reduce consumption of red meat, refined grains, and sweet foods and enjoy moderate consumption of dairy products, such as yogurt and cheeses.

Principle #2: Choose smaller portions and eat slowly enough to let your body tell you when to stop eating. Listen to your body.

How much food do you need to be satisfied? Well, your brain knows the answer to that question even if you don't. The problem is that while your brain is attempting to process the myriad satiety signals that determine when you should stop eating, you can easily swallow a few hundred (or thousand) more calories in the meantime. Portion control, combined with a slower pace of eating, will allow your brain more control of what (and how much) you consume.

The signals that tell us when we are hungry and when we are full are highly orchestrated. Believe it or not, our fat cells actually send signals to our brain in the form of the hormone leptin, which helps to decrease our intake of food. These leptin signals combine with signals coming from all along our digestive tract, including the insulin produced by our pancreas, to tell our brain that we are "full" or satiated. In fact, one of the reasons maintaining weight loss is often so difficult is that when people lose fat mass, they also lose a proportion of the leptin signals coming from those lost fat cells. In turn, their brain loses the satiety signals coming from leptin, which then may trigger a desire to eat more.

Taking more time as we sit and savor a meal, eating more slowly, has been shown to lower body weight by reducing calorie consumption. In one randomized study that compared the impact of slow versus quick eating rates on the development of satiation in thirty healthy women, slower rates of ingestion led to significant decreases in energy intake (by about 75 calories) while at the same time significantly increasing water intake. Even though the fast eaters consumed a higher number of calories, they were less satiated than those who consumed fewer calories eating slowly.[13]

Eating to the point of fullness or eating rapidly is tied to increased levels of metabolic risk factors.[14] One study of 422 men found that the body mass index (BMI) of those who ate quickly was significantly higher than the BMI of those who ate at a normal or slow rate. Researchers found the same was true in the women they studied.[15] Satiety signals are like traffic lights. If we drive as fast as possible, even when we see the signal change from green to yellow, we are unable to stop safely and often find ourselves crossing the intersection while the light is red. Is there a better way?

One of the results of slowing down to savor your meal is that you begin to respond to your body's own signals telling you to stop eating, a practice sometimes called "mindful eating." Defined in the literature as "an astute, non-judgmental awareness of the present moment," mindfulness is simply being deliberately aware of what your body is doing—a skill that can be learned fairly easily. Thus, instead of eating a meal on automatic mode, without awareness of what and how much is being consumed, mindfulness helps us pay closer attention to our food so that we notice the aroma, the taste, the texture, and the portion of the food being eaten. With greater awareness of how much is being ingested, we can respond more quickly to the light turning yellow and put the fork down before it turns red.

Portion Control

One of the most obvious effects of the abundance in Western culture is that we have become conditioned to desire more for less. From the "all-you-can-eat" buffets to the mega-grocery stores, we are on a constant hunt for the best food deals, most of which require us to "super-size" our portions to get the best bargains. As a result of increased competition and decreased food prices, portion sizes of foods have ballooned and now provide more energy (kcal) than the smaller portions served forty years ago, significantly contributing to the growing overweight and obesity problem. In fact, the average Americans' caloric intake grew from 1,900 calories in the late 1950s to a whopping 2,661 calories in 2008, with most of this increase occurring between 1970 and today.[16] The low cost of crops like corn, wheat, and soybeans has also made it easy for food companies to manufacture cheap, carbohydrate-rich food products with poor nutritive value, feeding the vicious cycle of increasing consumption. As a result, Americans today are forced to become more aware of and pay greater attention to portion sizes as a main factor in energy intake and weight management.[17,18]

Fortunately, what we actually put in our mouth is in our control, and studies have shown that one of the most profound ways to achieve and/or maintain a healthy weight is as simple as reducing the size of our portions. Simply put, when individuals are offered smaller portions, they eat less.[19,20] On the other hand, we might be able to take advantage of our desire for more, because when we are offered larger portions of healthy foods (like vegetables or fruit) we tend to consume more of them as well.[21] So it is important when developing a healthy eating pattern that we educate ourselves and our children in portion size and portion control.

Restaurants: The New Home Away from Home

In addition to the amount of food we eat, where and how we eat it also has a profound impact on our health and longevity. Now more than ever, Americans consume more food outside the home in a fast-paced lifestyle in which people rarely take the time to sit down to eat at their own dining room table. Research has shown that this fast-food lifestyle is linked with weight gain and a host of related chronic diseases.

The restaurant business is highly competitive. To compete with one another, restaurants seek to make foods that satisfy our tastes and our sense of value. To do this, they use a large amount of sugar, starch, saturated fat, and salt (do you want fries with that?). Estimating portion sizes without an accurate guide (which most restaurants are required to provide these days) is virtually impossible. Even after I became fairly good at estimating the calorie content of most common foods, I would routinely underestimate the number of calories of both appetizers and entrees when eating out, sometimes by as much as 400 calories!

When I grew up, eating out was a fairly rare occurrence. Today, however, eating away from home is much more common than than it was thirty or forty years ago (eating "take-out" at home doesn't count as a meal at home, by the way). I know some people who actually consume nearly every one of their meals in restaurants. Maintaining a healthy eating pattern with portion control becomes extremely difficult when consuming such a high number of meals away from home. If you travel often or find yourself eating at restaurants on a frequent basis, ask for the nutritional information or use your smartphone to look up the information online **before** you order. You might be saving yourself 400–800 calories in no time.

Principle #3: Unless purposely fasting, don't skip meals. Start each day with a balanced breakfast containing both protein and fiber.

When we talk about listening to our body in the context of eating slowly enough not to overeat, we also need to listen to our body telling us when we need to eat. This principle is straightforward, and the scientific literature is growing to confirm what our mothers have told us for centuries—breakfast is the most important meal of the day.

Skipping breakfast has become a national pastime. Various surveys suggest that between 10 and 45% of Americans routinely eat nothing for breakfast. The worst violators are 18–35-year-old males, while breakfast is routinely eaten the most amongst women over 65. This is an alarming trend that is not without consequence. As it turns out, there is a growing body of research showing that low breakfast frequency and quality are independent risk factors for both increases in weight gain and type 2 diabetes. Strong epidemiological data was recently published about a large cohort of non-diabetic men (29,206 healthcare providers), in whom researchers discovered that after adjusting for known risk factors, those who routinely skipped breakfast were 21% more likely to develop diabetes within a sixteen-year period of follow-up. While skipping breakfast and snacking through the day were both tied to increased BMI (a known risk factor for type 2 diabetes), the increased risk of 21% was independent of the change in BMI over these sixteen years.

Ideas to Help Control Portions

- Put your food on a plate instead of eating straight out of a large box or bag.
- Avoid eating mindlessly in front of the TV or while busy with other activities.
- Slow down! Eat slowly so your brain can get the message that your stomach is full.
- Take seconds of vegetables or salads instead of higher-fat, higher-calorie parts of a meal, such as meats or desserts.
- When preparing large amounts of food, freeze or store foods in portion-sized containers for later use.
- Ask for the nutritional information when eating out (check online—there's an app for that).
- Separate a portion of the meal before eating and ask for a take-home box.
- Before snacking, read the label for both **calories per serving and servings per container**.
- When you do have a treat like chips, cookies, or ice cream, eat only one serving, eat it slowly, and enjoy it!
- Avoid large beverages such as "supersize" soft drinks. They have an enormous number of calories.

The connection between skipping breakfast and negative outcomes has been especially studied in children, where increased obesity and lower school performance are routinely found.

This relationship has been studied in Asian countries as well, with a similar trend in obesity linked with skipping breakfast, suggesting that this dietary phenomenon is somewhat universal.[22] So what accounts for this phenomenon? If weight is basically a simple mathematical calculation between calories consumed and calories burned, why would skipping calories at breakfast actually increase our weight?

Ironically, it is often the same individuals who skip meals, especially breakfast, who later find themselves famished, justifying high-caloric, low-nutrient meals to satisfy their hunger. So, one of the straightforward answers appears to be that skipping meals tends to result in higher calories consumed and often poor food selection throughout the whole day. One of the other common explanations revolves around the idea that consuming calories early in the day increases the metabolic processes early, causing us to burn more calories throughout the day, whereas extended fasting into the late morning or early afternoon suppresses resting metabolic expenditures and triggers energy preservation mechanisms. While this theory is commonly cited, it has yet to be rigorously tested.[23]

My hypothesis is that, amongst other things, skipping breakfast on a chronic basis causes a disorder in the stress response system (we cover this in chapter 10). In short, as we awaken, the adrenal hormone cortisol is at its peak as a consequence of both the normal circadian rhythm and the process of waking itself. The sharp drop in cortisol that normally occurs in the hours after awakening is timed to occur with the expected consumption of foods, which should increase and stabilize blood sugar. In the absence of food intake, the body is forced to control blood sugar, in part, by maintaining higher levels of cortisol. Among other things, cortisol promotes insulin resistance, which results in increased fat-mass accumulation. Elevated cortisol also stimulates the signals to eat "comfort foods" that are high in salt, fat, and refined carbohydrates. Likely, all of these mechanisms—increased hunger, lower metabolic rate/energy expenditure, and cortisol-induced metabolic changes—account for the correlation between obesity and skipping breakfast.

But it is not just the skipping of breakfast that can harm us—what we eat for breakfast is also important. Numerous studies have shown that consuming a breakfast primarily composed of high glycemic carbohydrates (think of the typical free motel breakfast) will trigger a spike in glucose and insulin, which will rebound into low blood sugar, increased hunger, and increased consumption of calories throughout the rest of the day. One study even showed that eating this type of breakfast caused similar blood sugar effects as eating no breakfast at all.[24] Breakfasts lower in carbohydrates, with an additional emphasis on lower glycemic-index carbohydrates, create the best result in terms of glucose control after a meal.

The study I often cite when I teach about this concept is based on the single-meal effect of different types of breakfasts on obese teenagers.[25] In this study, twelve obese teenage boys were evaluated on three different occasions (cross-over design) and given a different breakfast each time. The three meals were equivalent in the number of calories (calibrated to 18.5% of each subject's resting metabolic rate) but differed in the glycemic index. The meals were either low glycemic index—cheese, spinach and tomato omelet, grapefruit, and apple slices (40% of energy from carbohydrates, 30% protein, 30% fat), medium glycemic index—steel-cut oats, milk, half & half, and fructose (64%, 16%, 20%), or high glycemic index—instant oatmeal, milk, half & half, and dextrose (64%, 16%, 20%). After consuming the meal, the teenagers had their blood drawn every thirty minutes to measure glucose and insulin levels; they were also asked about their hunger levels and were monitored to see how much food they consumed during the subsequent five hours.

Not surprisingly, blood glucose and insulin levels spiked the highest when they consumed the high glycemic-index breakfast. In fact, the total increase (measured as the area under the curve) after the high glycemic-index breakfast was twice as high as the medium glycemic-index breakfast and nearly four times higher than the low glycemic-index breakfast. As expected, the high glucose levels stimulated by the high glycemic-index breakfast led to the highest levels of insulin production, which pushed blood sugar levels below baseline within three hours after the meal. These events resulted in the teens' increased hunger, causing them to consume nearly twice as many calories over those five hours as they did when eating the low glycemic-index breakfast. Similar findings were observed in both obese and normal-weight preadolescent boys and girls (aged 9–12).[26] Different signals from food, different cellular outcomes.

If you routinely skip breakfast or are guilty of grabbing a donut and some OJ, you are working against your body's metabolic regulating signals. You might be saying, "Well, I am not hungry when I wake up, and shouldn't I listen to my body?" In this case, you might have to re-train your body or understand why, after eight or more hours of fasting, you are not hungry. You might have to start small (a few hundred calories) for a week or two, slowly shifting some of the day's total calories toward breakfast. Avoid high glycemic-index carbohydrates (donuts, bagels, juice); instead, choose foods with whole grain, high fiber, and modest protein levels. A balanced breakfast is part of a healthy eating pattern and should be included in your routine.

Principle #4: Eat real food! Limit your consumption of prepared and packaged products—and choose foods that would be familiar to folks 100 years ago.

-and-

Principle #5: Quality matters. Invest appropriately in your food selections; your life may depend on it.

These two principles are related to one another, so we will discuss them together. Both of these ideas require us to view food as an investment rather than merely an expense. In a world where the name of the game is getting the biggest bang for your buck, quality is often sacrificed at the expense of quantity. Investing just a bit more of your time and money in food preparation and food quality, however, can yield tremendous results when it comes to your long-term health. But just like investing time or money in any pursuit, the results take time to manifest.

When we say that you should "eat food," this might appear self-evident; of course, what else is there to eat? But if we look at what passes as "food" today, one might ask if our great-grandparents would recognize it as food. The need for convenience has pushed foods farther and farther from their natural state into processed and packaged consumables so that now a complete meal (with tray included) can go from the freezer to the microwave and then to the table in under three minutes. No preparation, no clean up, and everyone can choose a different meal. Is this progress?

It's no wonder we find it difficult to follow a healthy dietary pattern—we have very little connection to the foods we eat. Often, Americans don't know where (or how) their foods are grown, harvested, slaughtered, processed, packaged, or shipped, and until recently they haven't seemed to care. There are some promising signs that this is starting to change, as seen by the growing desire for organic foods, locally grown foods, and farmer's markets, and more scrutiny on food additives, trans-fatty acids, animal hormones, and genetically modified crops. Even so, we have a long way to go.

We know that most foods hold much more nutritional value when they are less processed, but this means that a bit more "processing" in the kitchen may be required. The nutritional value that you can add to a loaf of bread by grinding your own wheat and adding fresh-ground flaxseeds requires some basic knowledge and time. Going to the market or the co-op to find vegetables that have been grown without pesticides and herbicides and selecting them freshly ripened so they can be eaten raw or lightly cooked requires the investment of time and bit of extra cash. Every investment has a return, but what we often don't realize is that our lack of investment also has a return. The money and time we think we save by choosing cheaply prepared packaged foods will end up costing us much more in the long run as we use up years of time and money battling the health consequences of these decisions. Investing properly in quality food can help us avoid the greater cost of spending the last decades of our lives struggling with diseases that may have been prevented or delayed had we made better food choices before. If you believe that the foods you eat and how they are prepared contribute to your health (and by now you should), it is time to get serious enough to actually invest the time and energy to plan and prepare your own meals as much as possible. If you are a parent, get your children involved early; teach them how to prepare healthy foods for themselves—you will be investing in the health of your grandchildren.

Principle #6: Water should be your primary beverage; drink enough, and try to limit the number of liquid calories you consume.

Water is one of the quintessential nutrients of life and yet is often one of the most commonly neglected. Despite its great importance for nearly every bodily function, many of us are still at a loss when it comes to knowing how much we're supposed to drink each day and which other beverages count toward our daily needs. All this confusion about water needs comes as no surprise considering that the first official recommendation for adequate intake (AI) of water was only established in 2004 by the Institute of Medicine, coinciding with an increase in popular awareness about water needs for preventing conditions such as cancer, heart disease, and weight gain.[27] Prior to that, the RDA concluded that it was impossible to set a recommendation for water needs, and the National Research Council used a general rule of thumb of 1 ml/kcal (that would be two liters of water per 2000 calories consumed, if you're getting out your calculator).[28] Today's recommendations for daily water requirements, however, are based on national averages from the NHANES III data, although individual needs vary greatly. It's estimated that most of us need to get 80% of our daily hydration through beverages, mostly water, while about 20% of our hydration comes from the food we eat (less if you happen to avoid fresh fruits and vegetables).[28]

Throughout history, humans have relied on water as their primary source of hydration, struggling to ensure both an abundant and a clean source was available for their survival. Unfortunately, this struggle still exists in many locations around the world today. In the West, water abundance (at least for drinking) is rarely in jeopardy, and yet many choose other options. Countless individuals have replaced water with soft drinks to quench their thirst, and, as a result, sweetened beverages have become one of the major sources of calories in the American diet. Consumption of high fructose corn syrup, the major sweetener in commercial soft drinks, increased over 1000% between 1970 and 1990, and today, half of all Americans consume soft drinks every day. In fact, these beverages now constitute the leading source of added sugar in the average diet.[29,30] To make matters worse, the calories provided by soft drinks often fail to satisfy hunger the way solid food does, nor do they quench our thirst in the way water can, making sugary beverages a key player in the obesity epidemic.[30-33] If you want to maintain those good signals that your body is waiting for, limit the number of calories you consume through drinks.

So how much water should you drink per day? Well, that depends. How much you weigh (roughly 60% of that is water), how much water you lost recently to perspiration, and relative humidity will all affect the ultimate answer. The Institute of Medicine says that the adequate intake of total water per day is 3.7 liters for men and 2.7 liters for women.[†] The "8 by 8 rule" (8 glasses of 8 oz. each) equates to about 2 liters. Many rely on their thirst to tell them when to drink, and while it is true that most people's thirst and hunger mechanisms can help manage their net water balance, in many people the thirst mechanism is blunted and mild dehydration can set in well before their body tells them to drink. Others try to rely on the color and darkness of their urine as a gauge of hydration, but this is not always a reliable indicator of the need for water.[35]

So what's the bottom line when it comes to hydration and water?

- If you aren't already doing it, drink mostly water to keep yourself hydrated.

- Make sure your water source is clean and free of contaminants.

Common Sources of Liquid Calories

- Orange juice (8 oz.) – 134 cals
- Cola (12 oz.) – 151 cals
- Whole milk (8 oz.) – 146 cals
- Beer (12-oz. can) – 155 cals
- Red wine (5 oz.) – 125 cals
- Gatorade (8 oz.) – 63 cals
- Fruit punch (8 oz.) – 117 cals
- Fast-food chocolate shake (12 oz.) – 258 cals
- Starbucks Grande Cinnamon Dolce (16 oz.) – 240 cals
- Mango-peach V8 splash (8 oz.) – 80 cals
- Herbal tea (8 oz.) – 0 calories
- Red Bull (8 oz.) – 116 cals

---

† The AIs provided are for total water in temperate climates. All sources (according to IOM) can contribute to total water needs: beverages (including tea, coffee, juices, sodas, and drinking water) and moisture found in foods. Moisture in food accounts for about 20% of total water intake.

- Tea and coffee are fine for most people (in moderation); if the caffeine causes you to urinate frequently, consider offsetting this loss with additional water.
- Alcohol is dehydrating—plain and simple.
- Remember to include water-based soups and stews, herbal teas, and low-sugar fruit juices.
- Drink more water when you are physically active and when the weather turns hotter.

Principle #7: Be prepared for cravings that can jeopardize your plans for success.

Depending on where you are along your health journey, the principles we have laid out in this chapter may merely be great reminders of how powerful these simple steps can be or a monumental paradigm shift. If you fall into the latter camp, then there are certainly pitfalls around the corner that you can begin preparing for right now. Any change in our habits, especially eating habits, will be a struggle until a new "norm" has been established. Until then, the desire to revert back to those unhealthy patterns will sometimes overwhelm our best intentions. Ultimately, how you deal with these inevitable cravings is mostly dependent upon whether you anticipated them and adequately planned for them.

If you have already decided to choose a healthy eating pattern that guides most of what you eat (Principle #1), remember to remove from your cupboards, refrigerator, and freezer the foods that fall outside of the parameters of this new pattern. If you don't, they are likely to pull you back, like a tractor beam, into the old eating habits you are attempting to put behind you. One of the biggest culprits in our convenience-driven world is the ubiquitous and tempting "snack." Such a small and unassuming word—after all, it's just a snack, right?

By definition, snacks are foods consumed between meals, using the traditional three-meal-per-day pattern. The implication is that they are small amounts of food intended to "tide me over" until the next meal. The reality can be quite different. The snack business is quite competitive, and companies are all attempting to appeal to our urges and cravings (they know we love sugar, fat, and salt as well as strong flavors and colors). While few people would sit down to plan a meal consisting of caramel popcorn, beef jerky, sour balls, and a 32-oz. bottle of cola, there are vending machines with these items anywhere you might be looking for something to "tide you over."

Success doesn't mean abandoning snacks altogether; in fact, for many of us, appropriate snacking can help us maintain a more balanced blood sugar throughout the day. One study measuring weight loss success in post-menopausal women found that those who frequently consumed snacks in the morning were less likely to succeed in their weight loss and were more likely to have multiple snacks per day, while those who only snacked in the afternoon were more likely to eat fruits and vegetables (and succeed in their weight-loss goals).[36] While this study didn't make a direct analysis of the breakfast meals in comparison to the mid-morning snack, we know that mid-morning hunger is related to low satiety after breakfast (either skipping breakfast or consuming a high-glycemic breakfast will cause this) and food availability. It is highly recommended that you understand your own vulnerability to cravings (what, where, when, with whom) and plan to have healthy snack options (appropriate serving size) at hand for the occasion.

Healthy Snack Ideas

- Small handful of mixed almonds and walnuts (preferably unroasted)
- 1 handful assorted dried fruits such as dates, figs, or apricots
- 12–15 low-fat blue corn chips with ¼ cup salsa or guacamole
- ¼ cup hummus and ½ cup vegetable sticks
- 1 medium sliced apple with 1 T almond butter
- 1 low-fat cheese stick with whole grain crackers
- 2 brown rice cakes with tahini and jam spread
- Healthy protein bar (read label carefully)
- ½ cup celery sticks + 1 T peanut butter
- 1 hardboiled egg and ¼ cup carrot sticks
- ½ cup mixed berries and cherries
- 1 handful spiced dried green and chick peas
- 4–6 rye crackers and roasted vegetable dip
- 1 berry smoothie made with 6 oz. nut milk and ½ cup fruit and flax seeds

CHAPTER 9

A Life in Motion

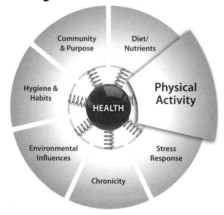

*"Leave all the afternoon for exercise and recreation,
which are as necessary as reading. I will rather say more
necessary because health is worth more than learning."*

—Thomas Jefferson (1743–1826)

JUST ABOUT EVERY STATISTIC we could cite tells us that populations living a Western pattern of life are less fit today than they were a century ago. Yet at the same time, the fitness level and athletic achievements amongst the most elite athletes in these same populations continue to improve almost every year. How ironic that every four years, millions of people camp out on their couches surrounded by junk food to watch the Olympics, wondering in amazement at the speed, strength, and flexibility of those on the screen. It is clear from the achievement of these athletes, from every possible ethnic background, that the physical limits and capacity of the human body are still being tested. The gulf between our physical potential and our physical fitness has never been wider.

Don't worry, we won't be trying to turn you into an Olympic athlete before the end of this chapter; there are other books better suited for that. We won't even be trying to give you a perfect workout guide to get into a swimsuit for summer. What we will do, however, is to lay out the basic principles that can help you reconnect the decisions you make about your physical activity to the signals your cells are waiting for.

Principle #1: Sedentary activity is an independent risk factor that can't be limited by exercise alone. Limit the time you sit uninterrupted at work, home, and everywhere in between.

Since the second half of the 20th century, physical activity has been known to be a cornerstone of health, essential for the prevention of chronic disease.[1-3] Over the last 100 years, however, our physical activity levels have been in a significant decline, due in large part to technological advances that have, quite simply, reduced our need to move. In the fifty years between 1950 and 2000, the percentage of sedentary occupations in the United States rose dramatically from 23 to 41%, and today American adults spend 50–60% of their waking day sedentary, in activities which do not increase energy expenditure substantially above the resting level (1–1.5 METS)—this means activities like sitting, lying down, watching TV, and other screen-based work and entertainment.[4] American children aged 6–11 spend six hours per day in these behaviors, while older adolescents (ages 16–19 years) and older adults (ages 60–85 years) spend nearly eight hours per day sedentary.[5]

So when exactly did we stop needing to move? Despite the fact that throughout history humans spent very little time sitting down, in today's automated world, most of our domestic and daily functions no longer require the expenditure of physical effort they once did. In contrast, almost all our day-to-day functions have become automated, including everything from transportation to house cleaning. In recent decades, researchers have taken a closer look at the effects of this increasingly sedentary lifestyle on our health, and much evidence is accumulating suggesting that excess sedentary time has a highly negative impact on health, independent of time spent physically active or exercising.[5] In fact, an increasing number of studies are showing that such a sedentary lifestyle contributes substantially to the morbidity and mortality of chronic diseases in the United States and in Westernized countries around the world.[5] Of the common sedentary behaviors, TV watching is the one most frequently linked with poor health outcomes. TV viewing, which far exceeds the time spent in any other leisure activity and represents the principal sedentary behavior in the U.S.,[6] has been connected repeatedly with obesity.[7] In the last few years, self-reported sitting time, TV time, and screen time have been linked with chronic disease and mortality.

The health hazards of sitting were first highlighted in the 1950s, when researchers found a two-fold increase in the risk of heart attacks in London bus drivers compared with subjects who were physically active.[8] By the 1990s, the accumulation of studies like the London bus driver study had shown that a sedentary lifestyle ranks only behind cigarette smoking and obesity as a key contributor to deaths from nine major chronic diseases, including heart disease, stroke, and cancer.[6] †
Sedentary lifestyles are estimated to account for approximately 23% of all deaths due to these chronic diseases and for 14% of all causes of death.[6] Sitting for long periods has additional consequences such as lower back and neck pain, deep-vein thrombosis, hemorrhoids, and both osteoarthritis and osteoporosis. As the field of research on the impact of sedentary activity has expanded, newer studies are clearly showing that a high amount of sedentary time is actually an independent risk factor for chronic disease, independent even from the amount of other physical activity you might do on a daily basis.[9,10] In other words, sedentary activity is not just the lack of something (exercise); it is the presence of something (sitting).

As we were putting this chapter together, one of the largest studies confirming the impact of sedentary activity was published. According to this large prospective study from Australia (222,497 people aged 45 years or older), death by any cause grows incrementally with the increasing number of daily hours spent sitting. This relationship was independent of sex, age, BMI categories, or even total physical activity level

---

† The most recent epidemiological studies now suggest that physical inactivity causes more deaths worldwide than tobacco.

among healthy participants.[11] This confirms what others have shown: that the amount of time spent being sedentary is independently associated with increased risk of weight gain, metabolic syndrome, diabetes, and heart disease regardless of hours spent being physically active.[5] In addition, sitting down for extended periods has been found to increase certain indicators of cancer risk, insulin resistance, inflammation, and body fat.[12,13] Simply put, sitting is a "signal" to our body that cannot be offset directly by exercise.

Sitting as a signal? Yes. In fact recent research suggests that when you place immature adipocytes (fat cells) under static pressure (similar to sitting), they mature more quickly and produce and accumulate more fat.[14] The mechanosensitive and mechanoresponsive activities of adipocytes, as the researchers call them, allow the cells to turn the static pressure on their surfaces into changes in gene expression and protein signaling which drive the changing metabolic activity. In other words, sitting can make you fatter.

We do know, however, that the health risks associated with sedentary behavior can be decreased significantly by breaking up prolonged sitting with short moments of activity. Interrupting sitting with short bouts of light- or moderate-intensity walking (two minutes, every twenty minutes) has been found to lower post-meal glucose and insulin levels in overweight/obese adults aged 45–65 years.[15]

So how much activity do you need to do to gain some benefit? As it turns out, some of the greatest benefits of physical activity result from the smallest increases from being sedentary to engaging in a minimal amount of physical activity. A prospective cohort study done in Taiwan explored the low end of the range.[16] Compared with inactive individuals, those in the low-volume activity group, who exercised for an average of ninety-two minutes per week (or just fifteen minutes a day) had a 14% reduced risk of all-cause mortality and a three-year longer life expectancy. The authors concluded that as little as fifteen minutes a day or ninety minutes a week of moderate-intensity exercise might be of benefit, even for individuals already at risk for cardiovascular disease.

Going one step further, a meta-analysis of thirty-three different studies examining the relationship between physical activity and risk of coronary heart disease (CHD) found that those who engaged in 150 minutes per week of moderate-intensity leisure-time physical activity had a 14% lower CHD risk than those reporting no leisure-time physical activity at all.[17] Those engaging in the equivalent of 300 minutes per week of moderate-intensity leisure-time physical activity had a 20% lower risk—and most of the benefit of risk reductions was gained by those first 150 minutes. Additionally, in the Nurses' Health Study, compared to people getting less than one hour of exercise per week (assigned a relative risk [RR] of 1), women who were active between one and two hours per week had an RR of 0.86 (multivariable adjusted, 14% reduction). In order to double that benefit, these women would need to exercise more than 3.5 hours per week (RR of 0.72, 28% reduction). By the way, we are not attempting to discourage high levels of exercise; we are merely trying to emphasize how beneficial those small increment increases can have when we move from being sedentary to engaging in modest daily activity.

Since research on the impact of sedentary time is still limited, there are no definitive recommendations or guidelines for how to break up your sedentary time. As a principle, however, you should consider taking regular breaks when you are sitting for long periods of time. At work, get up from your desk and stretch or walk around. Set your smartphone or computer calendar to remind you if you can't remember. At home, get up between chapters of your book or during television commercials to stretch or walk around. On a plane, get up and stretch. Driving your car, stop every couple of hours and walk around. Our principle holds true wherever you are—limit your extended sitting time for better health and a longer life.

Principle #2: Walking is one of the most fundamental of human activities and should be a regular part of each day when possible.

Over two thousand years ago, Hippocrates mused that "*man's best medicine is walking.*" Indeed, modern research has shown that his assertion may not be far from the truth, as it turns out that the health benefits of this simple and basic human activity are many. Walking is the most fundamental form of aerobic activity, and because it is a low-impact exercise that is also easy to perform, requiring no special equipment, it's a form of activity that almost anyone can engage in anytime, anywhere. As a testament to the dramatic lifestyle changes of the past few centuries, this most fundamental of human activities has moved from being a near necessity for most humans on the globe to an optional or even a leisure-time activity—one that is deemed important enough to study and for which we need to create guidelines.

You probably could have guessed that the more you walk, the more health benefits you get. A 2008 review of twenty-one publications found that longer walking duration, distance, energy expenditure, and pace were associated with a reduced risk of cardiovascular disease.[18] Remember the Diabetes Prevention Program we discussed earlier? They randomized 3234 pre-diabetic subjects to either placebo, metformin, or lifestyle modification to see which group would have the lowest incidence of diabetes over four years.[19] If you recall, the lifestyle group experienced nearly twice the preventative benefit as the group using the drug in those four years. What was that lifestyle intervention? Losing 7% of their weight and walking briskly for 150 minutes per week. It is partly due to the success of the DPP that this mark of 150 minutes of walking per week has become the standard goal for diabetes and cardiovascular prevention guidelines.

Another way to measure this goal would be to walk a total of ten miles per week. That amounts to 150 minutes of walking at 4 mph. This might be too fast for most people who are just getting started with their walking, so a bit more slowly (3 mph) is a good place to start. An easy way to think about getting this done is to pick a location exactly one mile from your starting point; then walk to that point and back for a total of two miles. Time yourself and try to accomplish this in at least forty minutes (3 mph), then increase your pace if possible. If you can do your two-mile walk five days per week, you have your ten miles and 150 minutes covered.

If you are completely sedentary and this sounds like too big of a jump, start slowly and gradually attempt to reach this goal over six months or so. Starting with short daily sessions of five to ten minutes each, build up to fifteen minutes twice a week, and then thirty to forty-five minutes of walking most days each week is a great way to slowly build walking into your daily routine. Set challenging but realistic goals for yourself; you don't need to do it all at once. Try counting your steps with a pedometer if you like; studies have confirmed the efficacy of pedometers in promoting physical activity in populations with high cardiometabolic risk.[20,21] If you have a smartphone, there are numerous free apps that will keep track of your walking time and distance (many by GPS) so you can see exactly how you are doing.[22]

When it comes to the time of day for your walks, some research shows that it may be beneficial to take your walk after eating a meal, especially in terms of lowering that post-meal rise in blood glucose level. Slow post-meal walking has been found to reduce blood glucose response to a carbohydrate-rich meal, and the magnitude of the benefit is directly related to the duration of walking.[23] Walking after an evening meal or over a lunch break at work may fit your schedule. If so, the walk might have a double benefit. Whatever it takes for you—a new pair of shoes, a walking companion, a change in schedule, or a different parking spot—walking might be your best medicine.

Principle #3: Consider a diverse exercise program involving cardiovascular activity and resistance activity if your goal is long-term chronic disease resistance, weight loss, and general fitness.

-and-

Principle #4: Intensity does matter— if you can kick it up a notch without hurting yourself, results can come more quickly.

We already know that when it comes to exercise, any amount of activity is better than none at all. Even low-intensity physical activity can decrease the likelihood of developing cardiometabolic diseases, especially when substituted for sedentary behavior.[21] A single bout of exercise can increase insulin sensitivity for up to sixteen hours in both healthy people and type 2 diabetics.[24,25] Since we already know the powerful impact of simply adding walking as a foundation to your physical activity, we want to explore how diversity and intensity can improve your health even further. The benefits of regular exercise or advanced physical activity extend beyond just weight loss and cardiometabolic risk reduction; exercise supports healthy psychological function, reduces depression, improves self-confidence and self-esteem, reduces mental stress, and facilitates cognitive performance.[26,27] Physical activity has also been found to attenuate markers of inflammation, the very process mediating most chronic diseases.[28] Who couldn't use some of these side effects?

The official recommendations of the American College of Sports Medicine suggest a combination of aerobic and resistance training, at a minimum of thirty minutes a day, five days a week, for general health. Aerobic activities include things like walking, running, biking, swimming, and dancing and may feature exercise equipment such as a treadmill, elliptical, stair-climber, and stationary bike. Until recently, the majority of research has focused almost exclusively on the cardiovascular benefits of these types of activities. We now know that resistance training has significant benefits that are independent of and additive to aerobic training. A form of strength training in which each effort is performed against an opposing force, resistance training supports the development of skeletal muscles and can provide significant functional benefits and improvement in overall health. Resistance training would include things like push-ups, sit-ups, squats, free weights, or weight machines.

Of course, there are other ways of getting both aerobic and resistance activities in your daily chores and recreation, like gardening, push-mowing your lawn, raking leaves, chopping wood, and engaging in a host of sporting activities. Listen to your body; it will tell you when you have exceeded your capacity. Be cautious when you feel pain or severe exhaustion; this might be time to rest a while.

The Signals Induced by Exercise

At this point, it shouldn't surprise you that what we call exercise or physical activity is interpreted by our cells as a number of biochemical signals. When we increase those signals by diversifying the types of physical activity we do, we enhance the cells' capacity to create a healthy outcome. This is especially true in the body's ability to manage blood glucose levels. When we neglect those signals (by being sedentary) or send the same signals over and over (lack of diversity), the cells attempt to rely upon other pathways to accomplish that balance, often depleting the buffering capacities of those other systems. In light of this, an increasing body of literature has shown us that resistance exercise, when added to aerobic activities, may be especially important in the management of type 2 diabetes.[29,30]

Remember when we discussed how insulin signaling triggers glucose transporters to move to the cell membrane to allow glucose into cells? We call that insulin-dependent glucose transport. As it turns out, within skeletal muscles, there are additional glucose transporters in similar transport vesicles that are induced, not by insulin, but by exercise alone. This is what we call insulin-independent glucose transport. And since 80–90% of glucose in the body is disposed of through skeletal muscles, stimulating these exercise-induced glucose transporters likely accounts for many of the additional benefits we see in the glucose management triggered by resistance exercise.[29] When researchers begin to look further at the genomic effects of exercise (some call this kinesiomics), we see even more signals are at work. Resistance training increases GLUT4 (the glucose transporter) mRNA in the skeletal muscle, allowing for more potential transport of glucose into the muscle, while being sedentary decreases GLUT4 mRNA levels.[31] Exercise also induces signals that drive gene expression to increase mitochondrial function, allowing for more efficient energy usage within muscle cells.[32] But the signals don't stop there. Recall how epigenetic changes can occur by modifying histones, the proteins upon which DNA is coiled in the nucleus. Researchers have now discovered that exercise actually affects histone modification, which allows, among other things, the GLUT4 gene to be more available for expression in muscle cells.[33] Some of these exercise-induced changes in muscle cell function are influenced by nutrient intake and can even be mimicked by certain phytonutrients like quercetin, resveratrol, and EGCG from green tea.[34] The cells are just waiting for the right signals in order to function properly.

Improving with Intervals of Intensity

Though the mechanisms for this effect are still being studied, it appears that high-intensity training induces greater reductions in abdominal obesity than lower-intensity, steady-state exercise.[35] Most guidelines consider seventy-five minutes of high-intensity exercise to be roughly equivalent to 150 minutes of brisk walking. If you are fit for such activity, high intensity can help you reach fitness and weight-loss goals more quickly. High-intensity exercise includes things like running, calisthenics, and cross-fit type training. Basically, it is any intense activity that can only be sustained for a relatively short period (requiring rests between bouts of training) and should produce a fair amount of sweat and heavy breathing. Obviously the level of intensity will grow as you become better trained; one person's warm up might be another's intense workout.

As it turns out, you don't necessarily have to choose between low-intensity and high-intensity training; you might benefit from short intervals of high intensity within a mostly low-intensity workout. This pattern is sometimes referred to as high-intensity interval training (HIIT). It might be as simple as taking your usual two-mile walk but finding four or five occasions to sprint for twenty to thirty seconds (or some specified distance). Since I live in the country, I will choose to sprint between two telephone poles, then walk for a bit, then repeat my sprint again five minutes or so later. I am usually winded after the sprint but fully recovered to sprint again just a few minutes later. Not only do I burn more calories and get a boost for my insulin sensitivity, I actually finish my walk faster this way.[36] Another way to incorporate intense training in a short period of time is to combine very intense bouts in rapid succession with short intervals of rest. Tabata training is one such method where twenty seconds of very intense activity (about as intense as you are able), perhaps jumping jacks or sprinting, is followed by ten seconds of rest. Eight rounds of this in four minutes (if you can make it) is a single exercise routine. Believe it or not, proteomic studies have been performed in rats to show changes in protein expression using Tabata-type training, including maximal GLUT4 expression.[37,38]

Variety Is the Spice of Life

One complaint that is often heard when it comes to exercise programs is that they are boring, particularly for those who choose a single exercise like treadmill walking. For the sake of both your mind and your body, you need to include variety in your routine. According to one cross-sectional study, increased variety of exercise equipment available to children, young adults, and older adults increased exercise participation and enjoyment without changing their perceived exertion: increasing the variety of exercise options will increase exercise adherence.[39]

Researchers actually studied this idea using three groups of men and women. Participants in the first two groups were asked to exercise three times per week for eight weeks and were given specific exercise guidelines; in the first group, the type of exercise was intentionally varied between workouts, while in the second group, members performed the same exercise at each workout. The third group had no set schedule, guidelines, or program to follow; they were given no instructions about varying their routine and had the freedom to do whatever exercises they wanted at each session. It turned out that the first group enjoyed their workout sessions 20% more than the members of the second group and 45% more than members of the third group. Among participants who stuck with the study through all eight weeks, the members of the first group were 15% more likely than the second group and 63% more likely than the third group to adhere to exercise on a regular basis. This study shows us two important factors: individuals enjoy their exercise more when they relate it to some program or goal, and variety of exercise will increase both enjoyment and compliance.[40]

A number of other benefits come with adding variety to our physical activity as well. Variety in exercise has been shown to reduce dementia; participating in a number of different activities may be even more important than frequency, intensity, and duration of physical activity with respect to dementia risk.[41] A study of a long-term, comprehensive, and diverse exercise program found that varying activities improved blood pressure, lipid and glucose metabolism, arterial stiffness, and balance in middle-aged and elderly Japanese.[42] Variety might also include changing the environment in which we exercise, especially if we can get outdoors. Some studies suggest that long-term adherence to exercise conducted in outdoor, natural environments or urban green spaces may be superior to that of indoor exercise interventions.[43] Another advantage of outdoor exercise is that it usually provides an opportunity for sunlight exposure that stimulates the skin to synthesize vitamin D.

Recommendations for optimal physical activity for preventing cardiometabolic disease include the following:

- Optimal physical activity should include a synergy of aerobic and resistance activities, both of which are important and provide their own benefits to health.

- Begin with moderate lifestyle physical activity and gradually increase intensity and duration.

- If you are new to exercise, use the national guideline of walking 150 minutes per week as a goal; work your way up to this amount over a six-month period if necessary.

- Aim to include resistance training twice a week (25%).

- Consider adding short, high-intensity intervals to your aerobic or resistance training for even more benefit.

- Revisit your current routine every few months for variety; explore fresh approaches to increasing the duration and intensity of your physical activity.

Principle #5: Posture matters; be mindful of maintaining correct posture and spinal alignment.

One of the additional side effects of our increasingly sedentary lifestyle is the hindrance of a healthy posture and proper spinal alignment. In the second half of the 20th century, chronic lower back pain has become one of the biggest public health problems among adults in the Western world.[44] The burden is a financial one as well, as data show that the costs of physician visits attributed to back pain in the U.S. have been increasing substantially.[44]

Attempting to link specific behaviors, even excessive sedentary behavior, with lower back pain has been difficult, as some studies have turned up non-statistical differences, while others have found clear evidence linking sustained sedentary work with lower back pain.[45] We know that the sitting position leads to an increase in disc pressure and increases strain on the lumbar spine and surrounding tissues.[45] According to one meta-analysis, those who are overweight or obese have an increased risk of lower back pain and seek more care for chronic back pain.[44,46] Of course this would make sense, as the additional weight would place increasing pressure upon the spine whether at rest or during movement. Practitioners of conventional medicine usually focus on the symptomatic reduction of pain, something that allows for a quick pharmaceutical solution. Rarely are they attempting to address the root problem of posture and proper alignment of the spine. Studies suggest, however, that addressing posture and physical alignment with therapies such as chiropractic care has been shown to be superior to medications for reducing sub-acute back pain.[47]

The chiropractic model[†] views posture as a type of biomechanical linkage, where any imbalances in symmetry or deviation from normal posture can promote mechanical, degenerative, and neurologic disorders.[48] After all, our spine houses most of the nerve signals that tell the rest of our organs and limbs when to function. If nerves that signal pain can travel to our brain when our spine is misaligned, this view proposes that nerve signals traveling from the brain to every organ in the body can equally be compromised when the spine is misaligned. Proper posture allows all the joints to be in a state of equilibrium (vertical and rotational forces balanced) with the least amount of physical energy being used to maintain the upright position.[49] When the body segments are out of optimal alignment for extended periods of time, the muscles adapt by either shortening or lengthening (depending on the position), leading to changes in nerve tissue and function.[50,51] Specific health conditions linked to poor posture in particular include scoliosis, headaches, dizziness, lower back problems, and impairment of the respiratory and circulatory systems.[52]

Here are some tips to help you maintain good posture and alignment:

- Check your posture throughout the day and correct back to neutral alignment as needed.

- Stay upright in your office chair—don't slouch. Get a new chair designed to maintain posture.

---

† Today there are numerous philosophies in the chiropractic world. Some rely heavily upon the view that misalignment of the spine (subluxation) accounts for symptoms beyond merely the traditional musculoskeletal pain and view realignment via chiropractic adjustment to be a fundamental therapy for a wide range of conditions.

- Get up and move—avoid sitting for longer than thirty to sixty minutes at a time.

- Create an ergonomic working environment. Think about the placement of your monitor, keyboard, and mouse to reduce strain. Use a foot rest to relieve lower back stress.

- Strengthen your core muscles in your back and abdomen—they will help hold proper posture and spinal alignment.

- Maintain good flexibility.

- Sleep on a good pillow and mattress. You spend 1/3 of your life on a mattress; it is worth the investment in time and money to find the right one for you.

- If you have chronic neck or back pain, consider a visit to a reputable chiropractic clinic.

Principle #6: Flexibility is critical—don't discount the benefits of stretching and low-impact exercise designed to improve circulation and flexibility.

The first thing we do every morning as we roll out of bed, almost by instinct, is to begin stretching our limbs. Even our dogs and cats love a good stretch when they get up. In fact, it is so natural to stretch we often overlook the fact that flexibility and activities that improve flexibility can send strong and healthy signals to the body.

Flexibility describes the total range of motion of a joint or group of joints. It obviously differs from person to person and from joint to joint, and it encompasses all components of the musculoskeletal system as well as specific neuromuscular pathways of the body.[53] Interest in flexibility training began just after World War I and increased in the 1950s, when people recognized that American children were unable to execute basic flexibility and muscular strength tasks successfully.[53] Today, this is a serious business where proper flexibility training includes coaches, personal trainers, fitness instructors, medical doctors, physical therapists, and health promotion specialists.

The physical benefits of stretching are many and include an increase in range of motion, reduction in the incidence and severity of injury, improvement in posture and muscle symmetry, reduction of lower back pain and injury, delay of muscular fatigue, prevention and ease of muscle soreness after exercise, and increases in the level of muscular efficiency and balance. Stretching exercises have also been shown to affect metabolic risk factors directly. In one randomized study of twenty-two males who were either at an increased risk for or already had type 2 diabetes, researchers found that one forty-minute session of passive stretching resulted in a significantly greater drop in blood glucose (compared to a "mock" stretching placebo).[54] Another study showed specific improvements in the fat hormone adiponectin and glucose homeostasis in subjects with cardiovascular disease after three months of practicing Tai Chi.[55] One review looked at the efficacy of a guided stretching program for lower back pain; five randomized controlled trials suggested that this therapy leads to a significantly greater reduction in lower back pain than usual care.[56] Additionally, low-impact exercise focusing on flexibility allows the participant to relax mentally, bringing to many an enjoyment they may not experience with more vigorous exercise programs.

While you can stretch anytime, anywhere—in your home, at work, in a hotel room, or at the park—you want to be sure to use proper technique. Stretching incorrectly can send the wrong sorts of signals to your body.

Some stretching tips:

- If you don't have time for even a quick exercise at work, stand often and stretch; bend your knees—this allows for hydration of the cartilage.
- Stretching is not the same as "warming up"; stretching cold muscles can result in injury. Warm up a little first, or stretch after your workout routine.
- Focus on major muscle groups and joint/ligament points.
- Avoid bouncing or quick stretching moves.
- Listen to your body—if it hurts, stop stretching.

Principle #7: Massage is real therapy and should be part of a healthy lifestyle.

Massage-like therapies are some of the most ancient and widely practiced modes of treatment recorded. Whether in applying healing ointments to the skin or as part of the physical therapy associated with the ancient bathhouse, massage has been a component of human healing for most of recorded history. Hippocrates even wrote that *"the physician must be experienced in many things, but assuredly in rubbing."*[57] In Chinese medicine, use of massage for healing dates back 4000 years, and it is still an important part of traditional Chinese medicine (TCM). I recall being told by Chinese medical students while I was in graduate school how they were required to massage a bag of rice until they had turned it into powder, apparently to strengthen their hands for therapies involving massage. Swedish massage was introduced to the U.S. in the 1850s, and by the end of the 19th century, the nation's first massage therapy clinic opened and a significant number of American doctors had added massage to their regimens.[58]

In the early 20th century, the rise of medical technology and prescription drugs began to overshadow massage therapy. For most of the 20th century, massage went out of favor as a medical treatment, with only a few therapists continuing to practice. In the 1970s, however, both the public and the medical profession began to take notice of massage therapy again, coinciding with a rebirth of a number of other "alternative" modalities. Today, more than 125,000 massage therapists practice in the U.S., providing 80 million massage therapy appointments every year.[58]

Massage and related body work therapies involve working and acting on the body with pressure, tension, motion, or vibration done manually or with mechanical aids. Target tissues may include muscles, tendons, ligaments, fascia, skin, joints, or other connective tissue, as well as lymphatic vessels or organs of the gastrointestinal system. There are over 250 types of massage and bodywork, including techniques as diverse as stroking, kneading, tapping, compression, vibration, rocking, friction, and pressure to the muscular structure or soft tissues. Some techniques are so soft you can't even feel them; others are so forceful you might need a week to recover.[57]

The benefits of massage therapy have been researched and are quite wide-ranging. Massage has been shown to reduce perceived stress in adults and infants, promoting sleep and relaxation.[41,42,59] Even without scientific proof, I think the anecdotal evidence is quite strong for correlating massage with a sense of relaxation; but of course there is data. A single 45-minute session of Swedish massage actually produces measurable changes in neuro-endocrine and immune function. When measured against "light-touch" as the placebo, Swedish massage improved measurements in the stress hormones ACTH and cortisol and modulated a number of circulating lymphocytes and mitogen-stimulated cytokine levels.[60]

How about one of our favorite targets, blood glucose control? Massage has even been found to impact blood glucose. In a randomized controlled trial in diabetic children, massage performed for fifteen minutes, three times a week, significantly reduced blood glucose levels in just three months.[61] As you will see in chapter 10, reducing perceived stress in diabetic and metabolic syndrome patients will create benefits well beyond what can be directly measured by the massage technique alone. As an investment in your health, consider massage therapy (by either a professional or a loved one) to be one of the many good signals that your body is designed to receive.

CHAPTER 10

Stress:
The Perception of Life

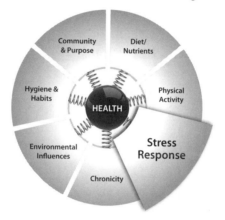

"If you ask what is the single most important key to longevity, I would have to say it is avoiding worry, stress and tension. And if you didn't ask me, I'd still have to say it."

—George Burns (1896–1996)

WHILE IT MAY SEEM obvious to most, the definition of "stress" has not been easily agreed upon by biologists over the past seventy-five years. Does stress define the necessary changes in adapting to a stressor, or the dysfunctions associated with failing to adapt to that stressor? When we think of stress, we most often think of negative stress, or, as some would say, "distress"; but positive events (wonderful surprises, passion, athletic competition) can elicit seemingly identical responses, from a physiological perspective. How much stress is "normal" or even necessary to maintain the stress response system, and how much stress is too much?

I have spent quite a few years studying the stress response system and the relationship of stress to chronic health. I am convinced that it is not only critical in our understanding of chronic disease management; it is perhaps the most neglected piece of the puzzle driving the pattern of metabolic diseases plaguing Western society today. It is for this reason I want to spend a little time giving an overview of the physiology of the stress response system before moving on to our principles.

Let's start with a bit of historical context. The scientist who is best known for bringing the concept of stress to the forefront of medical discussion is Hans Selye. His book *The Stress of Life*, written for the lay audience and published in 1956, popularized the notion of stress as the general response to a wide variety of insults.[1] He discovered in his research, mostly working with rats, that a recurring and consistent set of physiological outcomes occurred when animals were exposed to a variety of insults. He described these changes as hypertrophy (enlargement) of the adrenal gland, atrophy (shrinking) of the lymphatic organs, and ulcers in the stomach. Regardless of the insult—heat, cold, restraint, or pain—the physiological response appeared the same. It was almost as if all stress signals, irrespective of their origin, were translated through the same pathways.

He also discovered that each individual animal went through a predictable sequence of events when they were exposed to the same stress over and over. He named this sequence of events "the general adaptation syndrome" (G.A.S.). What he described is essentially this: animals respond very poorly upon the initiation of a stressor and, based on the intensity of that stressor, will suffer physiological harm; this he called the alarm reaction. He later found that under repeated "doses" of the same stressor, animals appeared to adapt or adjust their physiological response to the stress; he called this the stage of resistance. Finally, Selye observed that if the same stressor that had previously invoked resistance was continued on a long-term (chronic) basis, it would now exhaust the animal's ability to resist the stress and eventually could even kill the animal.

Even though Selye's model has simplified a very complex set of responses, his three-stage G.A.S. model is still the basis of much of the stress-related research to this day and is still used in helping to define the stages of human stress. In order to explain how stress impacts our health, we need to go just a bit deeper into the stress response system itself.[†]

The Stress Response System

The two primary areas involved in the stress response system are the brain and the adrenal glands. In the brain, the key focus for us will be the hypothalamus and the pituitary, which is why the stress-response system is often referred to as the hypothalamic-pituitary-adrenal (HPA) axis. Of course, the sympathetic nervous system (SNS), which can trigger our immediate fight or flight response, is also part of the stress response, and we will discuss this briefly as well. Let's look at what happens when we encounter a stressor.

All stressful events, whether they originate from outside the body (like getting a call from the IRS) or inside the body (inflammation from arthritis), send signals to the brain that are channeled through the hypothalamus. This small, almond-sized portion of the brain is actually made up of a number of nerve centers (nuclei) that monitor and control most of our bodily functions. The hypothalamus is tasked with converting all of these signals and translating them into hormone signals to

Selye's Stress Theory

1. The **alarm reaction**, involving increased adrenocortical secretion and activation of the sympathoadrenal system.
2. The **stage of resistance**, involving the balancing of the adrenocortical hormones' effect on water, electrolyte balance, and carbohydrate metabolism. The "true adaptation" to stress.
3. The **stage of exhaustion**, involving the depletion or exhaustion of the adrenal glands' ability to make corticosteroids.

Figure 10.1 **Selye's General Adaptation Syndrome**

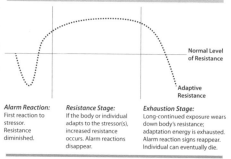

Normal Level of Resistance

Adaptive Resistance

Alarm Reaction: First reaction to stressor. Resistance diminished.

Resistance Stage: If the body or individual adapts to the stressor(s), increased resistance occurs. Alarm reactions disappear.

Exhaustion Stage: Long-continued exposure wears down body's resistance; adaptation energy is exhausted. Alarm reaction signs reappear. Individual can eventually die.

[†] For a full review of the role of the HPA axis, go to pointinstitute.org and check out the *Standard* [2010;9(2)].

direct the appropriate response of the body. The hypothalamus directs these processes, indirectly, by triggering hormones from the nearby pituitary gland. Together, the hypothalamus and pituitary control adrenal function, thyroid function, growth hormone production, male and female hormone function, kidney function, and much, much more.

When the hypothalamus is triggered by any stressor, it releases something called corticotropin-releasing hormone (CRH) into the pituitary gland, where it elicits both the production of adrenocorticotropin hormone (ACTH) from the posterior pituitary and the activation of the noradrenergic neurons. The noradrenergic system is primarily responsible for the immediate "fight or flight" response driven by epinephrine (adrenaline) and norepinephrine from one part of the adrenal gland (the medulla), while ACTH drives the production of the hormone cortisol from another part of the adrenal gland (the cortex). Under normal conditions, the production of CRH and ACTH fluctu-

Figure 10.2 **The HPA-axis and Stress Response System**

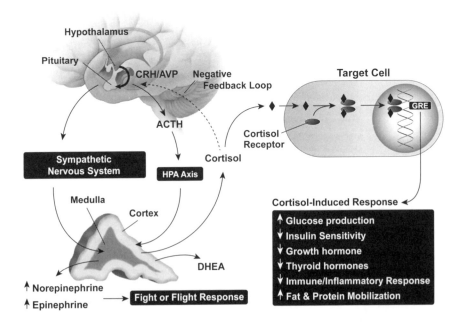

See text for details.

ates in a predictable circadian cycle and is controlled, in part, by a well-described negative feedback loop. When cortisol levels rise, it actually helps to reduce the levels of CRH and ACTH from the hypothalamus and pituitary, which functions to lower the cortisol production of the adrenal gland. It is the predictable rhythm and responses of the HPA axis that lend themselves to both experimental and clinical evaluation.

With such tight controls within our stress response system, it would seem that there is little room for error. Unfortunately, this simply isn't the case. As it turns out, the stress response system is very efficient at managing a relatively short-term stressful event (recall our story of being chased by a grizzly) but not so good when these stressors are unresolved and become chronic, as Hans Selye discovered in his animal experiments. The physiological changes that occur under stress, mostly as a result of increased cortisol secretion, are intended to help us get through the immediate needs of a stressful event. The stress response system is the ultimate in triage physiology, prioritizing the immediate needs, sometimes at the expense of long-term benefits.

Most popular discussions about the way stress affects our health invariably revolve around the adrenal gland. Often you will hear terms such as "adrenal fatigue" or "adrenal exhaustion" because cortisol is the most common metabolite measured in clinical and experimental models of stress, and cortisol is produced by the adrenal glands. It is assumed, then, that if we are measuring cortisol, we must be measuring adrenal function. This is only partially true. While it is clear that a large portion of the outcome of the stress response is mediated through the production and signaling mechanisms of cortisol, the emphasis should always be upon the whole HPA axis, primarily because most of the control and dysfunction of the stress response occurs outside the adrenal glands in the hypothalamus. Nonetheless, understanding the role of cortisol is vital if we are to learn how to combat outcomes driven by the stress response.

So what exactly does cortisol do? Well, first of all, cortisol is a steroid hormone within a class of compounds called glucocorticoids. These steroid hormones are powerful anti-inflammatory agents and, as their name implies, are also regulators of blood glucose. Like the stress response in general, cortisol is intended to shunt cellular activities away from long-term metabolic processes and toward those that function primarily for immediate survival and homeostasis, such as increasing available blood glucose, fats, and amino acids; increasing oxygen supply to tissue; and slowing long-term repair and immune functions.[†] These functions can be detrimental if maintained for too long, so the negative feedback loop that allows cortisol to limit its own secretion is actually designed to reduce long-term exposure of tissues to these short-term catabolic and immunosuppressive actions. Chronic and repeated stressors can lead to one or more forms of HPA axis dysregulation, which can then alter either the level of cortisol secretion or the cellular responses to cortisol.[2]

It is not surprising, then, that a host of chronic conditions are in one way or another associated with HPA axis dysfunction. As you can see from Figure 10.3 below, there are certain conditions that associate with an over-responsive HPA axis and another set of conditions that associate with an under-responsive HPA axis. We say "associate" because we don't always know if the HPA axis dysfunction is a direct cause or a result of the chronic condition. Most of the time it is a vicious cycle that makes it very difficult to decipher which dysfunction came first. Over a lifetime, a person can move from an over-responsive system to one that

Figure 10.3 **The Consequences of Stress Dysfunction**

Increased Activity of the HPA Axis	Decreased Activity of the HPA Axis
• Cushing syndrome	• Adrenal insufficiency
• Chronic stress	• Atypical/seasonal depression
• Melancholic depression	• Chronic fatigue syndrome
• Anorexia nervosa	• Fibromyalgia
• Obsessive-compulsive disorder	• Premenstrual tension syndrome
• Panic Disorder	• Climacteric depression
• Excessive exercise (obligate athleticism)	• Nicotine withdrawal
• Chronic, active alcoholism	• Following cessation of glucocorticoid therapy
• Alcohol and narcotic withdrawal	• Following Cushing syndrome cure
• Diabetes mellitus	• Following chronic stress
• Central obesity (metabolic syndrome)	• Postpartum period
• Post-traumatic stress disorder in children	• Adult post-traumatic stress disorder
• Hyperthyroidism	• Hyperthyroidism
• Pregnancy	• Rheumatoid arthritis
	• Asthma, eczema

Chrousos, G.P. (2009) Stress and disorders of the stress system
Nat Rev Endocrinal 2009 Jul;5(7):374-81

---

† More details about how cortisol drives the cellular response can be found in chapter 6. If you skipped that chapter because reading about genetics causes you stress, try it again after applying the principles listed in this chapter.

eventually is under-responsive, suffering from conditions in both categories. Recall that the hypothalamus is tasked with regulating almost every important function of the body. It is safe to say that the stress response system plays a role in nearly every chronic disease pathway and is therefore a fundamental part of any chronic disease management or recovery program.

So now that we have some idea about how the stress response system works and what can happen if it becomes dysfunctional, let's look at ways you can begin examining your own situation—what stresses you and what you can do about it.

Principle #1: Know what stresses you.

If you are going to be able to affect your own stress response, it is critical that you first know the most frequent sources of your stress, or at least what your brain thinks is stressful. We will focus on four categories of HPA-axis stress that can be measured and modified; they are glycemic dysregulation, sleep disturbances, chronic inflammation, and mental/emotional or perceived stress. Regardless of the outcome of stress upon the body, it is most likely that the root of the stress itself is derived from one of these four categories. Let's focus first upon the one most people think of when they think of stress.

No doubt, as a member of the "modern Western lifestyle" you could give several good descriptions of circumstances or individuals that "stress you out." You might, even now, be coming off a series of circumstances that have left you feeling like you have no way of handling one more stressful event. Perhaps you have been feeling burned out and exhausted for years and can't understand why it is hard to scrape up enough energy for the simple tasks of life. Whether you have a demanding job with constant pressure or are a graduate student in a competitive academic environment, a healthcare provider, a stay-at-home mom, or a retiree—your circumstances can often overwhelm your ability to cope, placing great pressure on your stress response mechanisms.[3]

Since the days of Selye, numerous researchers have attempted to discover the key elements that drive the brain's perception of stress. We say the brain's perception because unlike animals, the higher functions of the human brain allow us to perceive events differently, often with dramatically different responses. What researchers have discovered is that any event that moves us away from our pre-set expectations of life, whether the event is good or bad, is capable of triggering a stress response. Whether the event is current and real (an actual emergency or trauma), a memory of a past event, or even a hypothetical event (anxiety about a potential outcome), the stress response is surprisingly similar. The goal for the body, of course, is that the stress response should be short and designed to resolve the stressor. When we constantly trigger our stress response mechanisms with events that are not resolved, however, our response mechanisms begin to become disjointed, improperly regulated, and easily overwhelmed.

Scientists who have studied the features that cause some events to be perceived as stressful tell us that these events usually have four basic characteristics. First, events can trigger our stress response simply when they are **new** to us. The first time we do something, we anticipate how we might feel during that event (pleasure or pain), which triggers a stress response in anticipation. This doesn't mean that we should avoid events just because they are new. We may just need to adjust how we anticipate these events; perhaps getting more information about the event will reduce the stress response. When we combine a new event with **unpredictability**, the second feature of common stressors, we heighten the stress response. A simple example of this would be taking driving lessons for the first time on a busy freeway: stressful for the driver and the instructor or parent! Many people are stressed by their job simply because it is unpredictable. They have no way of anticipating what is coming and, therefore, feel a constant anxiety. The third characteristic of a stressful event is a sense of **threat**. This could be a threat to your physical well-being, but more often it is a threat to your psyche, your ego. If you are ever in a situation in which you think, "If I mess this up, what will they think of me?," then you can be sure your brain considers this a threatening and stressful situation. Public speaking is often listed as one of the most feared and stressful events (sometimes feared more than death) not because of an anticipated physical threat, but because of the potential threat to our ego. Lastly, common stressors typically cause the feeling that you have **lost control** over some situation. In some ways, this feature incorporates the other three characteristics as well. Mental/emotional stress is, in a word, losing control.

A perfect and common example combining these four stressful characteristics is experienced by a person who works at the middle-management level.[†] They feel the responsibility of performing new tasks (novelty) that typically have unpredictable outcomes while at the same time threatening their job approval. Rarely are the middle managers in control of the outcome measurement they will be judged upon (their bosses dictate this); and as managers they cannot completely control

Consider Testing Your Stress Response System

The level and timing of the adrenal hormones, cortisol, and DHEA (dehydroepiandrosterone) produced throughout a given day can be a good predictor of the stress response in most individuals. Measuring both cortisol and DHEA levels is a common tool for many clinicians to help assess what level and type of stress you are experiencing (DHEA-S, the sulfated form of DHEA, is also a common laboratory measurement). These hormones can be measured from blood, urine, or saliva samples. The advantages of using salivary measurements include the fact that collection is fairly non-invasive, samples can be collected anytime and anywhere (especially good for measuring circadian rhythm), and sample collection does not create a stress response (needles!).[4]

Most often, salivary samples are collected four times throughout a "normal" day: once upon rising, once in mid-late morning, once in the afternoon, and once before bedtime. Clinicians will be looking for the total levels of cortisol and DHEA and the proper diurnal rhythm. Some clinicians will use laboratories that will also measure additional hormones such as melatonin (in the bedtime sample) and sometimes even testosterone and estrogen. These other hormone levels can identify certain related conditions to help define a better treatment approach.

Through a process of physical examination, health history, lifestyle assessment, and functional testing, you can work with your clinician to find out what level and type of HPA axis stress you are currently experiencing and develop a specific plan for helping you recover.

---

† Sonia Lupien, the director of the Centre for Studies on Human Stress in Montreal, described these as N.U.T.S.: Novelty, Unpredictability, Threats, Sense (of loss of control).

the outcome (they must work through those they manage). This combination is the perfect recipe for stress. Not surprisingly, middle managers are considered to have the highest stress in most corporations, leading to high rates of turn-over, burnout, and poor job satisfaction.

If you're going to begin to get your stress response system in order, you really need to know what is stressing you or what your brain perceives as a stressor. Additionally, consider what components (novelty, unpredictability, threat, loss of control) make that particular event or relationship the most stressful; perhaps you can think of ways to respond differently. As we explore this further, remember that it is our *perception* of the event or circumstance that really drives most of the stress—not the event itself.

Principle #2: Take control of your stress response.

Now that you have some idea of what might be driving your stress response system, you can begin doing something about it. Simply put, if stress is a lack of control, then reducing stress means we must feel like we have regained some of that control. Below we will list a few of the most common things you should consider in the evaluation and management of your stress response.

Take Control of Your Health

One of the greatest worries people have is about their own health. Often people experience aches and pains that they do little about, hoping they will go away, perhaps afraid to find out if they might be something serious. Since nearly every chronic ache and pain, or any chronic condition, for that matter, is likely to involve some sort of inflammation, the stress response system is already activated.

We have already mentioned that cortisol is one of the body's best anti-inflammatory agents. Synthetic corticosteroids have been created to help combat major injuries and inflammatory diseases; these cortisol-like drugs are some of the most potent available for reducing inflammation. So when we have any inflammatory process going on in the body, the signals reach the brain as powerful HPA-axis triggers driving elevated cortisol production. These signals might be coming from arthritis, a chronic inflammatory bowel condition, gum disease, food or airborne allergies, chronic sinusitis, even obesity. In fact, if you suffer from any condition ending in "itis," you are likely sending regular signals to your stress response system, slowly depleting its metabolic reserve.

It is critical to discover the root cause of any chronic health issue you might be suffering so you can slowly remove the signals triggering your stress response system. Depending on how serious the condition is, augmented lifestyle intervention strategies are likely to be the most helpful. Adjusting your eating pattern (hopefully based on the Mediterranean diet) to include foods and dietary supplements that are anti-inflammatory in nature is likely to be a helpful place to start. It is difficult to repair or support the functions of the HPA axis if there is an uncontrolled inflammatory process in the body, so you must take control of this the best way you can.

Take Control of Your Physical Activity

Since we already covered the principles of physical activity in chapter 9, we will be brief in our discussion here. We just want to remind you that physical activity is important for proper health and proper stress management. In the right balance, it helps maintain insulin sensitivity, blood glucose, muscle mass, and body chemicals (endorphins) that can relax us. People who feel stressed tend to be more sedentary and less likely to be physically active—be careful that you don't get into this vicious cycle.

On the other hand, strenuous training can add stress to our bodies. In fact, rigorous training for triathlons or marathons is actually a clinical model for HPA axis stress, for which interventions are being tested on a regular basis.[5] So even if you skipped the last chapter because you are an athlete and are already highly trained, realize that you may be vulnerable to stress-induced illnesses when you over-train. If you are routinely exhausted hours or days after exercising, your body may be telling you that your stress response system has lost some of its metabolic reserve. A proper incorporation of light exercise that includes stretching is ideal for producing the health benefits that result from stress reduction.

Take Control of Your Work

When most people think of stress, they define it as "too much to do and not enough time to do it." Perhaps this describes every day at your current job. Remember the middle managers we described earlier; stress is highest when we are given responsibility (and accountability) without feeling like we have the tools (authority, finances, time, skills, etc.) to accomplish the task. Does this sound like your job? Does this sound like one of your employees?

Stress isn't for middle managers alone. We have all seen the pictures of various American presidents at the beginning and end of their terms. Four or eight years often seem to age them twenty or thirty years. The weight of responsibility is stressful—you need to decide how much you can handle and choose your job/career accordingly. You must ask yourself if the amount of stress at your workplace is overwhelming you and how much of this could be relieved. Think about the four traits of common stressors. How can you eliminate the stress of novelty, unpredictability, threatening events, and loss of control? Speak with your co-workers or supervisor about the need for adequate warning when new changes are coming or for additional training when new skills are required. Ask for more specifics about what is expected of you so you can feel more control over your job performance. If all else fails, consider other employment options. With few exceptions, there is no job worth losing your health. If you think this is financially impossible, you may need to create a plan to make the transition slowly.

Reducing Your Stress at Work

- Don't skip meals and breaks to get more done; you need proper nutrition to combat stress.
- Resolve issues with supervisors and co-workers as soon as possible.
- Recognize the things that are truly under your control, and don't fret about the rest.
- Re-organize your work surroundings for better efficiency.
- Use an organizer to plan your day—your mind stresses when it thinks you will forget something; write it down.
- Get new skills or training if needed to perform up to expectations.
- Schedule as much vacation as you are allotted—and ask for more!

Take Control of Your Finances

Are you financially stressed? Do you worry about money or bills regularly? Do you feel guilty spending money for non-necessities? Do you limit your recreation time or vacations due to lack of finances? If so, financial pressure may be a major stressor in your life.

It goes without saying: financial instability creates tremendous anxiety and stress. It can cause major friction in a marriage and bring constant worry. While this book is no place to give financial advice, finding a competent advisor to help you eliminate your debt and create a plan for financial stability will result in more peace than you can imagine. Debt is not always about the lack of money, but usually about the lack of proper priorities. Financial stress is no respecter of income; it reaches both ends of the socio-economic ladder. As we strive for the things we think will bring us pleasure before we can afford to pay for them, those very things can become our nemesis once the overdue bills arrive. If you have found yourself nodding or cringing as you read this, perhaps you have discovered that this may be a place to start. Seek out a credible financial consultant (there are many free services available) to help you evaluate your financial situation and design a program to give you financial control once again.

Take Control of Your R&R

If life's enjoyments seem like a thing of the past and you find yourself wishing you could go back to the day when you had no stress, then you definitely need some R&R. You need to find a place where you can feel relaxed enough to allow yourself to rejuvenate. It should be the opposite of our four stress characteristics. That is, it should be familiar (rather than new), it should be predictable (no surprises), it should be without threat (and guilt-free), and it should be a place where you are truly in control. You need times like this frequently (even daily) but also for extended periods of time.

Schedule a fifteen-minute break every afternoon where you can brew a cup of tea, turn off your computer monitor and cell phone, turn on some music that soothes you, and...*just relax*. Schedule a massage once a month and budget this as a health expense. Write down a list of things that you really find guilt-free pleasure enjoying and begin finding ways to add them back into your schedule. Finally, take a real vacation. By this I mean taking a vacation where you can really break free from the normal stresses of your daily routines, where you are both relaxed and engaged in other activities. This is important enough that in the next chapter we will explore the "science" of a good vacation.

Take Control of Your Relationships

There is no doubt that some of the greatest pleasures and some of the worst experiences in life involve relationships. Few things can lift our spirits like being with someone we love; few things can damage our spirits more than a relationship full of tension and strife. Below are some simple things you might want to consider to help reduce the stress, or increase the blessing, of relationships.

Make a list/Make a call

Write down a list of the people you enjoy being with. Maybe you have a personal phone book or keep such a list online. When was that last time you saw or spoke with these people? I don't mean just checking their Facebook page for updates or even posting a comment on their blog, but actually sitting across the table or talking on the phone? Make a point of calling or seeing these people more often—you will be surprised how good you will feel once you do. Don't worry about how long it's been; they will love the surprise.

Thank someone

Being thankful and expressing your appreciation for those who help you in any way is therapeutic. When we fail to express genuine thanks to those around us, we build up a mental "debt of gratitude" that weighs on our minds until it is paid. Sometimes this is more difficult with those we see every day—our coworkers, our spouses, our children, our parents—but these are the people who need to hear it the most, and these are the relationships that affect us the most. Have you ever tried writing down all your blessings, all the things you can be thankful about? Try it, and you will be amazed at how your perspective changes from stressed to blessed.

Resolve your disputes

Relationships will eventually produce conflict, some minor, some major. Conflict in a relationship can be extremely stressful and often results in drastic turmoil in the lives of many people. Often the issue seems to get worse the longer it is left unresolved, turning a minor misunderstanding into a major dispute. If you dread the thought of running into someone because of an unresolved dispute, your hypothalamus would really like it if you decided to resolve your conflict.

Again, make a list of individuals you need to resolve disputes with and prioritize them from the smallest dispute to the largest (if this requires a spreadsheet, see a counselor). Try resolving the smallest one first. This will probably be easier than you think, but you might want to get a friend to help out if it is appropriate. Once you get the first one out of the way, move to the next one on the list. Not only will it get easier each time, but the relief you will feel from the previous resolution will spur you on to get through the list. Not everyone will want to resolve the conflict, but even in those situations, you will have much less stress knowing that you attempted an honest resolution.

Forgiveness

Forgiving is certainly related to the above topic of resolving conflicts but deserves its own heading. Often there are persons who genuinely hurt us physically, mentally, or emotionally. Regardless of the offense, the unwillingness to forgive them causes bitterness, resentment, and anger when we think of them or the events they caused. If the list you made above includes someone you are unwilling to forgive, you may want to consider seeking out a spiritual leader or counselor to help you work through the issues involved. Conversely, if you have wronged someone and do not feel forgiven, consider going to that person and asking for forgiveness and reconciliation. The release of guilt and the sense of relief will do wonders for your soul and your level of stress.

Principle #3: Get off the glycemic roller-coaster.

While we covered diet in quite a bit of detail already, this is such an important principle related to the stress response we must re-emphasize it in this chapter. As we mentioned earlier, one of the most stressful events on the body is glycemic dysregulation, the constant fluctuations in blood glucose caused by poor glucose regulation. Low blood sugar is a major stressor for the brain, triggering the HPA-axis response to produce cortisol, which in turn stimulates cells to begin producing more glucose to combat the hypoglycemia.[6] While this is important after a night's sleep and one of the reasons that cortisol is normally high upon waking, we don't want to use the stress response to regulate our bad eating habits throughout the day.

When we eat foods high in refined carbohydrates (sweets, unrefined sugars, high glycemic-index foods), our blood sugar rises quickly, causing insulin production from our pancreas to spike in response. This overproduction of insulin helps to push glucose into cells quickly, causing blood glucose levels to drop down rapidly, often resulting in a lower than optimal blood sugar level for a short period of time. This low blood sugar event usually occurs soon after lunch, when we feel sleepy and would like to take a quick nap. At this point, our cortisol levels kick in due to the hypoglycemic stress, and our body begins the process of moving us back to a normal blood glucose level, which might take thirty to forty-five minutes. We often don't or can't wait for this process to bring us back to normal blood glucose levels; instead we routinely self-medicate with some type of chocolate or caffeine (or both), attempting to shake off that drowsy feeling. For some, this cycle of glycemic stress comes once or twice every day, placing a constant burden on the stress response system.

Controlling glycemic response is critical to help reduce chronic stress. Choosing foods that promote glycemic stability is a foundation to the lifestyle changes that will reduce stress. Foods with low glycemic index and high soluble fiber will help ease the insulin spike that drives blood glucose below normal. Breakfast is especially important. Eating a breakfast with proper glycemic balance that includes good sources of both protein and fat will start you off right. In addition, eating more fruits and vegetables will help reduce inflammation, a common burden to the stress response system. Consuming higher amounts of omega-3 fatty acids (fish, fish oil, flaxseeds, green leafy vegetables) and reducing omega-6 fatty acids (most other oils except canola and olive) will also promote appropriate stress responses.

It is difficult to overemphasize the importance of maintaining balanced blood sugar throughout the day. Using your diet and physical activity, rather than the HPA axis, to manage your blood sugar will go a long way toward protecting the metabolic reserve of your stress response system. Obesity, inflammation, and unhealthy eating patterns are directly linked to both the causes and effects of stress and should be at the forefront of concerns for both clinician and patient alike. When you are stressed, you naturally reach for unhealthy foods loaded with fat, salt, and sugar—junk foods and so-called comfort foods.[7] Animal studies actually show that the stress hormones are down-regulated when animals are fed "comfort-food" meals.[8] It appears that our body attempts to "medicate" our stress response with foods that end up driving more obesity, hypertension, diabetes, and heart disease.[9] Stress and disordered eating patterns are a vicious cycle that drives a host of metabolic disorders; they must be tackled together.[10]

Principle #4: Without proper sleep, repair of the stress response will always be limited.

Sleep is your body's way of resetting itself metabolically and psychologically. We are designed to function optimally on a twenty-four-hour circadian rhythm. Sleep is what helps our body readjust to the stresses we place upon it during the day. If we are not getting the appropriate amount of sleep or we keep adjusting our sleeping pattern (day shift to night shift, etc.), it prevents our natural stress response from functioning properly. Like glycemic dysregulation, it is impossible to overemphasize the role of sleep and chronicity in the control of the HPA axis and the repair of the stress response. In fact, this subject is so critical to our overall health that it is a separate sphere within the Lifestyle Synergy Model, one we will cover in chapter 11.

One of the things that I always remind clinicians of when they discuss a patient's stress profile with me (based on salivary cortisol testing—see sidebar on page 189) is to notice the rhythmic nature of the cortisol curve. If they are lacking a normal circadian rhythm, very often there is some disturbance in the sleep pattern of the individual. I always tell them that while dietary supplements and other stress-reducing therapies will be helpful in decreasing some of the symptoms of stress, it is virtually impossible to make major changes in the HPA axis without improvements in the sleeping pattern of the patient. Sleep is that powerful. I feel confident in saying that it is virtually impossible to be healthy if you do not have a healthy sleeping pattern.

It is my opinion that recognizing and managing the stress response system can be one of the most potent avenues to preventing and reversing chronic disease. You can see how the metabolic disease pattern, with its attending chronic inflammation and glycemic dysregulation, coupled with the growing perception of stress and related sleeping disorders, all comes crashing down upon the stress response system. If you are suffering from any chronic condition and are serious about getting better, you need to begin taking control of the things that control you. You need to rebuild a strong stress response system.

CHAPTER 11

What Time Is It? How the "Clock" Rules Your Life

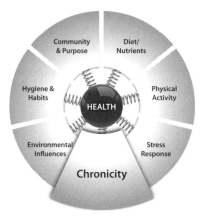

There is an appointed time for everything.
And there is a time for every event under heaven—
A time to give birth and a time to die;
A time to plant and a time to uproot what is planted.
A time to kill and a time to heal;
A time to tear down and a time to build up.
A time to weep and a time to laugh;
A time to mourn and a time to dance.
A time to throw stones and a time to gather stones;
A time to embrace and a time to shun embracing.
A time to search and a time to give up as lost;
A time to keep and a time to throw away.
A time to tear apart and a time to sew together;
A time to be silent and a time to speak.
A time to love and a time to hate;
A time for war and a time for peace.

—Ecclesiastes 3:1–8

THE FIRST SUMMER AFTER I moved to our forty-acre property in Central Wisconsin, I began to explore it on a regular basis. As an amateur naturalist, I hoped to catalog each type of tree, shrub, and plant on my property by genus and species. That summer I also attended my first botanical medicine conference in the hills outside of Asheville, North Carolina, after which I was even more enthusiastic to find out whether I had any medicinal plants growing just around my home. I returned from the conference in early June and was a bit disappointed. I found yarrow, mullein, and a few more obscure medicinal plants; but at that time in the mid 1990s, the herb St. John's wort was popular, and since it was basically a weed, I thought for sure I would have plenty growing somewhere on my acreage. Alas, it was not to be—or so I thought at the time.

You see, St. John's wort doesn't bloom until just about the day of St. John—June 24. When the end of June arrived, the small green plants that I had initially overlooked suddenly bloomed into clusters of small yellow flowers that oozed a reddish, flavonoid-rich juice when squeezed. They were, like a weed, everywhere. So now every year, almost exactly on June 24, St. John's wort dots our landscape for most of the summer.

Since most of my excursions around my property took place in the evening after returning home from work, you can imagine my surprise one weekend morning when I discovered dozens and dozens of dazzling purple flowers just down the hill from my home. How could I have walked by these beautiful specimens evening after evening without ever even noticing them? By happenstance, it turned out that these flowers were another type of "wort," this time Spiderwort.† What I soon learned was that Spiderwort flowers open up in the morning, revealing three deep purple petals, and close up again before the heat of the afternoon. Each individual flower on a plant opens for just one or two days. I discovered when I cut a few plants to bring in for a bouquet that for about three days individual flowers still maintained their circadian

---

† There are numerous plants whose common English name contains "wort," which is derived from an Old English/Germanic term meaning "plant" or "root," often related to plants with medicinal benefits. Other than St. John's wort (*Hypericum perforatum*) and Spiderwort (*Tradescantia spp*), my property contains Motherwort (*Leonurus cardiaca*) and Figwort (*Scrophularia nodosa*); but I never did finish cataloguing all the plants so there might be more.

cycle, opening in the morning, then closing in the afternoon. After about three days the cycle ended.

Those who study the details of botany could unfold in painful detail how plants of all sorts are programmed to respond to daily (circadian), day length (seasonal), and perhaps even monthly (lunar) rhythms.[†] What most people don't often think about is how powerful these same signals are for human biology and human health. The study of how time-keeping mechanisms affect living systems—called, appropriately, chronobiology—is turning out to be a critical piece of the puzzle to answer our drift toward chronic disease.

Chronobiology—A Short Excursion

While our fascination with "time" goes back as far as we can study human behavior, the scientific study we call chronobiology is relatively recent, being established as a discrete discipline by Pittendrigh and Aschoff in the 1950s.[1] Using observations recorded in both plants and animals of all types, scientists have linked the most basic biological functions (feeding, reproductive activities, migration, etc.) with various intervals of time. From these studies it became obvious that there were two general phenomena keeping biological systems in sync with various cycles of time: those which appeared to be internal to the organism (an internal "clock") and those which were external to the organism but influenced the organism's internal clock.

When organisms that appear to follow a strict twenty-four-hour circadian cycle are moved to a location where there is no change in light (always light or always dark) and no change in temperature, they will drift a bit from their strict twenty-four-hour cycle. The internal pacemaker of the organism, as we will see in a moment, is programmed to oscillate in a fashion that approximates the daily cycle, usually somewhere between twenty-three and twenty-five hours, depending on the organism. In order to stay on pace, the organism must synchronize with some external cue from the environment in a process called entrainment. Chronobiologists often use the German word "zeitgeber," which

---

† While gardeners from antiquity to modernity have espoused the belief that certain plants respond to lunar cycles or gravitational influence and promote "planting by the moon," many researchers are unconvinced there is proof of such an influence.

means "time-giver," to describe an entraining agent or synchronizer. The most obvious zeitgeber is sunlight, which is considered one of the most powerful synchronizing signals for the broadest range of organisms, from blue-green algae to humans. Cycles of different lengths have other zeitgebers, such as circalunar cycles (monthly) synchronized by the moon, circannual cycles (yearly) synchronized by day length, and circaseptan cycles (seven days) with an as yet unknown zeitgeber.

These outward timing devices (sun and moon), along with their relationship to the astronomical constellations, have been used as "clocks" in a literal sense for all of human history.† From the sundial to the smartphone, humans have always wanted to know what time it is. Whether it was the need to understand when to anticipate the annual migration of a particular animal for hunting purposes, when certain plants should be harvested, or when your tribe was getting together for the next celebration (or simply when dinner would be served), knowing the time was vitally important. The accuracy and precision of time-keeping devices in antiquity based upon these three zeitgebers is truly astonishing. But this chapter is not about ancient time-keeping devices. Instead, I want to discuss something that is, in my opinion, even more astonishing—the time-keeping devices within our bodies.

The Clock Within

We saw from the last chapter how the stress response system is tightly integrated with circadian rhythm. As it turns out, the part of the brain that consolidates all stress signals and coordinates its response, the hypothalamus, also houses the center of the body's internal clock. Within the many nerve bundles (nuclei) that make up the hypothalamus is a group of tightly packed neurons called the suprachiasmic nucleus (SCN). Light signals travel from the retina through the optic nerve and combine with counter-regulatory signals from the pineal gland (which makes melatonin) in the SCN to help synchronize our circadian cycle. By means of neuronal signals and hormone signals (through the pitu-

---

† Even the biblical account of the creation of the sun and moon and stars (Gen. 1:14) says that they were put in the heavens as time keepers *"to separate the day from the night, and let them be for signs and for seasons and for days and years."*

itary), this pacemaker portion of the hypothalamus sends signals to the whole body that entrain each cell's biological rhythm.

We have already discussed in detail one of those signaling mechanisms, the production of CRH in the hypothalamus which causes ACTH secretion from the pituitary to eventually trigger the adrenal glands to produce cortisol (see chapter 10 for details). The circadian nature of this cycle is a classic feature we now know is enhanced by access to light in the morning. This feature of the HPA axis is called the cortisol awakening response (CAR) and represents the highest peak of cortisol throughout the day. Without some form of oscillation between light and darkness, entrainment of the SCN is hindered. When experiments attempt to define the free-running circadian cycle present in humans, independent of the influence of light/dark signals, we are told that it is about 24.3 hours. What this tells us is that the majority of the circadian rhythm is programmed in the SCN itself, but external signals are still required to fine-tune the clock on a regular basis. When we remove or choose to change the timing of those expected signals, we begin to stretch the physiological resilience of the cellular pathways and feedback loops that tightly control our biological rhythm.

While circadian control of our sleep/wake cycle is an obvious example, what is often not appreciated is that a large percentage of all our cellular activities follows a circadian pattern.[†] Metabolism of lipids and carbohydrates, release of numerous hormones, blood pressure, body temperature, immune system activity, bone turnover, and mental acuity are just some of the many physiological areas regulated by circadian rhythms.[2] Just consider the powerful regulatory effects of cortisol alone; all the gene expression induced or repressed by this powerful steroid hormone, which follows a strong circadian fluctuation, will be influenced in the same rhythmic fashion. In the same way, the expression of myriad other genes and their resulting metabolic consequences is being controlled by other pathways, each operating in a circadian fashion.

---

† While the most commonly cited statistic is that between 10–15% of all genes are controlled by circadian signals, there are some researchers who argue that there is data to suggest that nearly 100% of gene regulation is influenced by circadian oscillation in some way or another.

What has been discovered over the past decade or so is that there is a tight interplay, via complex cellular feedback loops, between the circadian cycle and metabolic function. Specific to our discussion here, there is a high degree of circadian control upon those metabolic functions that control blood sugar, glucose metabolism, insulin function, and adipose physiology.[3] Circadian disruption of different sorts has now been linked with numerous metabolic diseases such as obesity, metabolic syndrome, cardiovascular disease, diabetes, and hypertension.[4] Likewise, acute events such as heart attacks, strokes, and hypertensive crises tend to peak at certain times of the day, suggesting both an immediate and a chronic impact of circadian influence.[5] Even subtle shifts may be detectable. One study in Sweden reported a small but statistically higher incidence of acute myocardial infarction (AMI) the week after the spring daylight savings time adjustment (which shortens the day), which was not seen with the fall time adjustment (which lengthens the day).[6]

With such wide-ranging circadian control of so many metabolic functions influencing every organ system in our body, it seems quite implausible that all of these functions could be controlled only by the SCN/hypothalamus sending circadian signals to each and every cell. While electrical impulses within neurons are very fast, the other signaling molecules require more time and are constrained by enzyme degradation, hormone-binding proteins, receptor binding, cellular diffusion, and a host of other factors. Could it be that each cell has its own clock mechanism, and the SCN is merely the inner "zeitgeber" acting as the master synchronizing agent?

Prior to the 1990s, scientists had already discovered specific proteins and genes that regulated circadian biology in simpler organisms like yeast and fruit flies. When it came to the more complex mammalian models, they designed experiments using mice that were given a chemical to cause mutations in random genes, then they looked for circadian disruption in the offspring of these animals. By placing those offspring into dark chambers, they discovered a mutant with a free-cycling circadian shift from the normal 23.5 hours of the wild-type mouse to one that cycled at 27 hours or longer depending on whether it had one (heterozygous) or both (homozygous) mutant genes. When the researchers found the gene responsible for this change they named it *Clock,* and the protein encoded from this gene they called CLOCK.[†] The nuances describing all the other proteins that have been discovered to be a part of the intracellular circadian controlling mechanism are not necessary to make our point. Needless to say, it involves no less than a dozen major proteins/genes—most of which regulate each other in a series of transcriptional feedback loops. The result is like a chemical pendulum that swings on a nearly twenty-four-hour cycle. And just as light can help fine-tune the master clock in the SCN, so the signals sent from the SCN to tissues and cells throughout the body help synchronize each cell's circadian and metabolic machinery. Research has now even revealed specific miRNA sequences that are triggered by light with epigenetic influence on gene expression.[7] Like an orchestra, where precise timing turns thousands of different notes into beautiful symphonic sounds, so each cell and organ system maintains exquisitely-timed processes that control the mystery of metabolism.

Hey, Buddy, What Time Is It?

The discovery of circadian-controlled gene expression (chronogenomics) and epigenetic modification in just the past few years has blossomed into a whole new area of research and is beginning to challenge the results of many previous studies. Imagine if you were researching how a particular protein or gene is up-regulated or down-regulated (or unchanged) in an animal when given a particular substance, but you were unaware of the circadian fluctuations and controls of the proteins and genes you were measuring. Without knowing, you might have collected some of your data in the morning, other data in the evening—after all, it really didn't matter, you surmised. Now you can see that it is very possible you could have missed a real change in gene expression or mistakenly thought all changes were caused by your test substance rather than normal circadian fluctuations. A reassessment of a host of metabolic processes is likely going to be necessary, changing the way we understand cellular function from the standpoint of chronobiology.

---

† It is common to use capital letters to denote the protein and lower-case italics to denote the gene that encodes the protein. In this case, since mutants in this protein/gene combination disrupted the circadian rhythm, CLOCK stands for circadian locomotor output cycles kaput; who says scientists have no sense of humor?

Now that I have made you all budding chronobiologists, you are probably wondering what you can do to improve your health with all this knowledge. Hopefully, I have impressed upon you how important biological rhythms are to nearly every function in your body; so obviously your health is going to suffer if you make decisions that alter these basic time signals. Decisions like quickly traveling across multiple time zones (jet lag), inadequate sleep durations or consistency, working nights or swing shifts, limiting your access to sunlight, and taking hormones like birth-control pills† are just a few of the signals you control when it comes to maintaining your biological rhythms. The principles we have outlined for this sphere of our Lifestyle Synergy Model are designed to create strong and consistent rhythmic signals to promote an optimal metabolic foundation.

Principle #1: Sleep is the body's great reset button. You cannot be healthy without appropriate sleep.

We introduced this topic in the last chapter because of the strong inter-relationship between the stress response system and circadian rhythm. We can now see how these powerful signals control nearly every facet of our physiology. It is difficult to overestimate how important sleep, both quantity and quality, can be to maintain your health and protect you from chronic disease. If you have ever suffered from insomnia or any other sleep disturbance, you know how lack of sleep can affect your mood, your energy, your eating habits, your ability to fight off infections, your libido, and just about everything else. And you're certainly not alone. Statistics show that around 50–70 million Americans suffer from some sleep disorder, and 10% routinely use some form of sleep medication. Add to these statistics the ongoing trend of shortened sleep duration, and we can see how circadian signals have been radically altered in humans over the past few generations.

I don't know how many times I have heard someone say that they wish there was a pill that could substitute for their need for sleep. Sleep,

---

† Researchers in chronobiology have mainly focused on the daily cycle, whereas the monthly cycle, most prominently featured in the menstrual cycle of pre-menopausal women, is another biological rhythm managed quite significantly by hypothalamus and pituitary signaling.

to them, appears as just an inconvenience that prevents getting more things accomplished. On the contrary, if life is a steady rhythm of signals, ebbing and flowing between activity and quiescence, sleep is the body's way of reorganizing all of those signals while you are too preoccupied (sleeping) to mess things up. You will spend more time sleeping than doing any other single activity in your life. Think of it this way: sleep is so important it is designed to consume 1/3 of your existence. This is not a coincidence, and there is no substitute.

As we showed in the beginning chapters of this book, one of the trends that has occurred in the U.S. population over the past few centuries is a one- to two-hour reduction in the average sleep time.[8] Epidemiologists have linked these changes in sleep duration with numerous metabolic diseases such as obesity, type 2 diabetes, hypertension, and cardiovascular disease, as well as hormones and metabolic precursors for these conditions.[9-13] Sleep is even powerful enough to modify genetic risk for some of these diseases. In a study of twins performed in the U.S., the genetic predisposition for obesity (measured by BMI) was increased in those twins who achieved less than seven hours of sleep per night but was dramatically reduced in those getting more than nine hours of sleep per night (genetic heritability of BMI differed two-fold between these groups).[14] Since these twins had similar genes and environments, the level of influence of these two hours of extra sleep per night is quite staggering, but not surprising. Sleep is one of the most powerful metabolic regulators we currently have—and it has a dose-response curve!

Short sleep duration is now also linked with difficulty in achieving weight loss, even in studies that severely reduce caloric intake and increase physical activity.[15] What researchers have discovered is that sleep-induced influence appears to follow the classic "U-shaped curve" we discussed in chapter 7. That is, risk appears to be linked with either too little or too much sleep time, and the lowest risk appears to be associated with adults who achieve between seven and eight hours of sleep per night.

But these effects require years and years of shortened sleep, right? Well, not really. Several studies suggest that changes in insulin sensitivity and glucose regulation might occur each and every time you deprive yourself of adequate sleep, likely compounding the effect on your body's metabolic machinery. In one particular study, ten overweight, non-smoking adults underwent fourteen days of moderate calorie reduction, where they were assigned to either 5.5 hours or 8.5 hours in bed.[16] While they only achieved an actual sleep difference of about two hours between the two groups (7.25 vs. 5.15 hours), the researchers discovered an interesting difference in metabolic function based on sleep duration. Both groups lost a similar amount of weight (~3 kg), but the group getting less sleep lost less of that weight as fat (by 40%) and more of that weight as fat-free mass (60%). Not surprisingly, the body composition changes resulted in the resting metabolic rate (RMR) being significantly lower in the group getting less sleep, which would translate to difficulties in preventing weight re-gain in the future.

If we look at a few studies that are even shorter in length, we see that we don't need to wait two weeks to see these changes. In one particular study of fifteen healthy normal-weight men, just two consecutive nights of shortened sleep duration (going to sleep at 2:45 AM rather than 10:45 PM, both times waking at 7:00 AM) had significant negative impacts on glucose and insulin levels after the breakfast meal.[17] So just two nights of shortened sleep duration can demonstrably impact our insulin sensitivity. There are even studies that show changes in satiety-signaling hormones, stress hormones, and metabolism with a single night of shortened sleep duration.[18,19]

While it may be difficult to avoid a night of shortened sleep now and again, it is clear that pulling an "all-nighter" to study for finals may carry with it some metabolic consequences. But our self-induced sleep deprivation is a national pastime, and we often celebrate it with gusto. For example, one of the radio stations in the small city near my home, Stevens Point, Wisconsin, hosts the largest trivia contest in the world every spring.[†] The contest begins on a Friday afternoon and doesn't end until Sunday evening, fifty-four blood-shot hours later. This turns out to be an annual experiment in the combined effects of sleep depriva-

---

† 2012 was the 43rd year of the trivia contest, which is now streamed online for groups around the world. If you are interested in doing your own sleep-deprivation study by joining along, their website is http://90fmtrivia.org/. As an undergraduate student during the pre-Internet era in 1989, I participated in the 48-hour version of this contest.

tion, extended sedentary time, mental stress, and junk food cuisine—a potent combination indeed. I'm sure we could all name a few events like this one that incorporate sleep deprivation as a mandatory component. Most of these are planned and prepared by high school or college students long before they realize their metabolic reserve won't last forever.

I have two general recommendations for your health concerning sleep duration. Avoid, if possible, getting less than six hours of sleep on any given night (minimum seven or eight hours). If you cannot avoid it, or choose to get less than six hours of sleep, then at least avoid eating foods that will exacerbate your glycemic response during breakfast. Depriving yourself of adequate sleep is a stress signal that increases your vulnerability to glucose dysregulation; you can diminish the long-term impact of this event by avoiding high-glycemic foods and choosing balanced meals with protein and fiber to minimize this effect.[†]

What's Keeping You Up at Night?

We recommend that you target and prepare your schedule to get eight hours of sleep per night, with as much of that coming before midnight as possible. Listen to your body; it will tell you when to sleep—unless it is medicated to avoid these signals (caffeine, sugar, etc.). Here is a list of things you should consider as you try to figure out how to get adequate amounts and better quality of sleep.

- Are there other medical conditions waking you up at night? Prostate issues, lower back pain, restless leg syndrome, hot flashes/ night sweats, anxiety, and many other conditions can make it difficult to fall asleep or stay asleep. If you have any condition that is making it impossible for you to get a good night's sleep, it may be creating more of a problem than you think. See a healthcare professional if necessary, but resolve this issue as soon as possible.

- Prescription sleeping medications are rarely a good solution for your sleep problems. Recent research confirms a very troubling increased risk of all-cause mortality and cancer in those who take

---

† *The Circadian Prescription* by Sid Baker, M.D., describes a dietary approach to control circadian living. While the Lifestyle Synergy approach differs in many ways from his approach, there is much to commend about his focus on this issue.

prescription sleep medication.[20] They found that the top third of sleeping-pill users had greater than a five-times higher risk of death and a 35% higher risk of cancer. There is a debate about whether these drugs are the cause of the higher risk or if the culprit is chronic insomnia, which is coincident with the use of these drugs. Either way, the use of hypnotics to induce sleep is not the signal the body is looking for to maintain rhythmic balance. If you are taking prescription medication to help you sleep, work with your physician to see if you can find solutions to end your need for these drugs.

- Avoid caffeine in the evening. Not only will caffeine delay your ability to fall asleep, but for many it acts as a diuretic agent, increasing the need to urinate late at night. If you get up frequently at night to urinate, consider reducing your consumption of all beverages in the evening hours.

- Is your bedroom set up for perfect sleep? Avoid watching television or working on the computer while in bed, as this will delay your sleep. How about your mattress, your pillow, your sheets? Are they helping or hurting your cause? Think about the shades on the window or any lights that could be bright enough to affect your sleep (from computers, clocks, etc.).

- Does your sleeping partner snore? If they are interrupting your sleep, get them some help so you can get some sleep.

- Do you snore or have sleep apnea? This is a major sleep disturbance that has been directly linked with increased risk for numerous cardiometabolic outcomes and is highly correlated with obesity. If you have been told that you snore or often feel like you are unrested even after "sleeping all night," you may have sleep apnea. This is not something to ignore. See your clinician for a diagnosis of sleep apnea so you can begin addressing this issue right away.

- Are you on a restricted carbohydrate diet? Some of you may be taking the dietary principles in chapter 8 to heart and reducing your glycemic impact. In the zeal to reduce carbohydrates, some individuals go to bed with very low blood sugar, which can cause a stress response in the middle of the night, triggering a rise in cortisol levels, resulting in shorter sleep duration. Consider adding a small, balanced snack before bedtime.

- Too much exercise in the evening can also make it difficult to get to sleep. If you can only get your physical activity later in the evening, consider toning down the intensity. On the other hand, being sedentary is also a hindrance to good sleep, so don't use this as an excuse to skip your workout altogether.

- Have you had your melatonin levels checked? Melatonin is a key hormonal signal for proper sleep, and your levels can be measured with a simple saliva test in the evening before bedtime. Ask your clinician about ways to supplement melatonin if you are low.

- Do you have low progesterone levels? Perimenopausal women will see a decline in progesterone levels often years before estrogen levels decline. This drop in progesterone can often lead to difficulty sleeping. Ask your clinician about ways of testing and treating low progesterone levels.

Principle #2: Sunlight is critical for circadian control. Maintain contact with sunlight as often as possible.

In our modern world of artificial lighting, the day/night cycle that is supposed to regulate our circadian rhythm is no longer driven by the sun alone. Numerous animal and human studies show that the circadian rhythm can be shifted inappropriately by the use of artificial light/dark cycles. At the same time, a particular form of depression called seasonal affective disorder (SAD) appears to be very clearly linked with reduced access to regular sunlight, which is exacerbated in northern latitudes in winter.[21] No matter how you look at it, human beings are intended to get adequate and regular sunlight to maintain proper circadian recalibration.

Since we will cover other aspects of sun exposure in the next chapter (vitamin D, etc.), we have just a few simple suggestions to improve your circadian rhythm using sun exposure. When you wake up in the morning, use sunlight to expose your body to light. Open the curtains and let the sun shine in. If you routinely wake up before sunrise, use low-level lighting rather than bright lights until the sun rises. The same is true in the evening; use low-level lighting after the sun has set to begin preparing your body to produce melatonin, which will help you sleep. If you use sunglasses routinely, wait a few minutes while in the sun to allow your eyes to properly interface with the sunlight before putting them on (unless you are coming into the sunlight in the morning from working the night shift—see below).

Principle #3: Beware the phase-shifters: jet lag, shift work, and night shift.

Modern life has contributed to the opportunity for regular and sometimes abrupt circadian phase-shifting activities. One of those events is jet lag, which wasn't really possible until humans could cross multiple east/west time zones as quickly as we can today with jet travel (jet lag is not experienced when traveling north and south). Jet lag, or experimental phase-shifts that mimic jet lag, affects animals as well as humans. Researchers using experimental jet lag conditions of a single, multi-hour shift in the day/night cycle have shown that this shift causes alterations in gene expression and metabolic function within the SCN. They have discovered that repeated phase-shifting is more harmful in females, as estrogen appears to influence clock-related gene expression in the SCN as well as in peripheral tissue. This estrogen/circadian interaction is thought to be the link between jet lag (and shift work) and both reproductive issues and breast cancer risk for female subjects.[22]

From an experimental perspective, individuals who change working shifts on a regular basis (shift work) experience a sort of repeated circadian "jet lag."[23] Individuals who are subject to shift work are at a higher risk for obesity, metabolic syndrome, diabetes, and cardiovascular disease, much of it attributed to the diminished circadian regulation of their metabolism.[24-27] In animals subjected to similar experimental conditions, chronic phase-shifting leads to changes in circadian gene expression as well as changes within the SCN and a decrease in neurogenesis within the hippocampus, the center of our memory.[28] When humans are put into an experimental circadian shift with reduced sleep duration (to mimic shift work), they experience lower resting metabolic rates and changes in insulin responses to meals, which recover only after nine days of re-training to normal circadian rhythm. Unfortunately, individuals may work odd shifts and only have a few days to recover before the next set of phase-shifting labor begins. By constantly changing the signals intended to maintain our body's metabolic rhythm, shift work stretches the physiological resilience of the cells much more quickly, resulting in the metabolic consequences we see in these subjects.

Finally, there is the night shift or third shift. Here we have an individual who is attempting to be active at the time the body is designed to sleep and sleep when the body is designed to be active. Study after study has shown that alertness, no matter how many years someone has been acclimated to night shift, is lower during the night than during the day. The link between the night shift and some of the more notable accidents involving human error has not gone without notice; Chernobyl, Three-Mile Island, the *Exxon Valdez*, the *Titanic*, and Bhopal are just a few. Not surprisingly, individuals who work the night shift are similarly at increased risk for all chronic diseases, especially the metabolic diseases we have been discussing: obesity, metabolic syndrome, diabetes, and cardiovascular disease.[29-32]

My first suggestion is simply to be aware of how these phase-shifting activities can harm your health. If you experience jet lag now and again, it is unlikely to have a major impact if you are aware of the tendency toward insulin resistance and therefore choose low glycemic-impact foods as you are adjusting. Most "treatments" for jet lag involve circadian synchronization using sunlight, extra sleep (on the plane), melatonin, and diet. If jet lag is extremely common for you, extra effort should be made to maintain healthy signals from as many of the other Lifestyle Synergy spheres as possible to expand the buffering capacity that maintains your resilience against chronic diseases.

If you are an employer, ask yourself if you can manage your business without needing to run during the night hours. Investing in extra equipment and inventory may be inexpensive compared to the potential errors and long-term health damage effects on your employees. If you are employed on the night shift or in a job that requires constant deprivation of sleep or changes in sleeping pattern, your health is being compromised. You should consider ways of getting on a day shift position, even if it means changing employers or changing careers. In the meantime, be aware of how your body is designed to use sunlight. When you leave your shift in the morning, use sunglasses (blue-blockers) to avoid direct sunlight contact with your eyes while traveling home. This will at least prevent your body from attempting to readjust before you sleep, which has been shown to lengthen sleep time in night shift workers.[33] You are still phase-shifted, which becomes a dilemma on the weekend, but it will allow you to sleep better and be more alert on the next night shift.

Principle #4: There is nothing wrong with a little nap or sleeping longer on the weekend; it will help, but it won't substitute for regular sleep of seven to eight hours per night.

No matter how you add it up, most Americans are depriving themselves of much-needed sleep on a regular basis. We can try to hide it with caffeine and sugar all we want, but the urge to sleep will often hit us in an afternoon lull or on the long commute home. What scientists call "sleep debt" is thought of like a bank account; the less we put in, the larger the amount of debt. What is still being debated is whether we can pay back our sleep debt with large quantities of sleep on vacations, weekends, or naps.

The major discrepancy in determining the answer to this question is in the objective short-term versus long-term effects of sleep debt and payback sleep. Alertness/sleepiness are the easiest to measure, and the evidence suggests that napping has a proven track record.[34,35] In general, short naps improve alertness and energy levels whether a person recorded a sleep deficit the night before taking the nap or not. Studies suggest that naps must be at least ten minutes to give a consistent benefit, but naps longer than thirty minutes will often result in sleep inertia, where the person may not fully realize the benefit of the nap until the sleepiness wears off. The best timing for the nap (morning or afternoon) is a bit more difficult to pinpoint, but it appears to be most beneficial between 2 and 5 PM, when the alertness level is typically the lowest in most people. For most of the year, mid to late afternoon coincides with the hottest part of the day, which, not surprisingly, is the least active time of the day for most animal species as well. If you are in a situation where a ten- to thirty-minute nap is possible, taking it during this time-frame might be a real benefit to you.

Whether you can pay back your sleep debt by sleeping longer on the weekend is a bit more challenging to prove. This has been looked at in a few cases, mostly as it pertains to long-term sleeping patterns in school-age children and young adults.[36] In a population of school children in Hong Kong, researchers found that children who slept the least during the school week had a higher likelihood of being overweight but were even more at risk if they didn't get catch-up sleep on holidays and weekends.[37] The best advice at this point is for you to listen to your body; it will usually tell you when you should just turn over and catch up on a little more sleep.

Principle #5: Seasons change, and so do you. Adjust yourself as best you can to the changing seasons for optimal lifestyle signals.

As we discussed earlier in this chapter, human activity was previously influenced quite profoundly by the changing seasons—the circannual rhythm. Before refrigeration and long-term food storage, diet was constantly affected by seasonal variation in available foods. Springtime provided green vegetation, summer brought certain vegetables and berries, while fall allowed for an abundance of fruits, nuts, and tubers that could be stored for winter. As the length of daylight changed, our access to sunlight and our expenditure of energy also changed.

Today, however, our routine can be identical nearly every day of the year. We can eat the same foods and keep to the same schedule regardless of the changing seasons. The consequence of ignoring seasonality is not easily decipherable, as there are numerous other events that correspond to seasonality, including signals that drive the length of the life cycle of certain cells.[38,39] Since the master controlling signals of the circannual cycle are thought to involve the hypothalamus, anything that negatively influences the circadian rhythm is likely to also affect the circannual cycle as well.[40]

In general, I recommend increasing your awareness of how your activities could be adjusted to better follow seasonality. Eating more foods grown locally, wherever you live, will allow your diet to follow a certain seasonality. Eating more food when you are more active (summer) and less when you are less active (winter) is another healthy pattern. Sleeping longer in the winter months and getting some amount of daily sunlight throughout the whole year will help your hypothalamus adjust to the changing day length. Even attending seasonal social gatherings (holidays) and vacations can act as important zeitgebers for your circannual rhythm.

Principle # 6: Your body is designed to have regular rest every week and throughout the year. Make your weekends and vacations count.

In the U.S. especially, people are judged by what they can accomplish; and even though we revel in our leisure-time activity, ironically, Americans don't cease from their activities very often. We are among the top workaholics in the world. According to a survey by the National Life Insurance Company, four out of ten employees state that their jobs are "very" or "extremely" stressful, and those in higher-stress jobs are three times more likely than others to suffer from stress-related medical conditions and are twice as likely to quit. Women, in particular, report high levels of stress related to conflict between work and family.[41] To

Figure 11.1 Vacation Days Earned and Taken in Different Nations

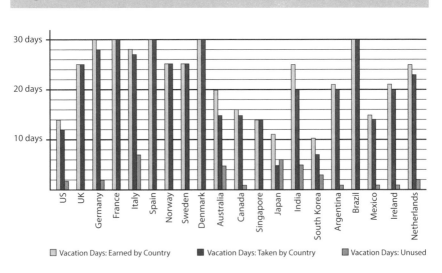

☐ Vacation Days: Earned by Country   ■ Vacation Days: Taken by Country   ☐ Vacation Days: Unused

Note that most of the nations in Europe allow almost twice as much vacation as the US, resulting in almost 3 times more vacation days taken. [43]

make matters worse, in 2011, American workers forfeited $34.3 billion worth of hard-earned vacation days.[42] Without sufficient restful and restorative getaways, all that stress and hard work are certain to damage our health and limit the pleasure of our productivity.

Taking a respite from the routine of life has its roots in the Sabbath. As the oldest prescription for stress relief, this involves taking one day per week of complete rest, providing us with much-needed replenishment physically, emotionally, mentally, and spiritually. But is there more behind this seven-day cycle of labor and rest than meets the eye? I believe there is.

As it turns out, scientists have discovered another rhythm in animals and plants that cycles at approximately seven days; we call this a circaseptan rhythm.[†] They have discovered a number of human functions that appear to follow this circaseptan rhythm, such as immune function, heart rate, blood pressure, mental function, and mood.[44–46] While many of these fluctuations are subtle, they are detectable, and there is even data to suggest a weekly pattern in deaths from specific causes, such as cardiovascular events on a Monday.[47] Some transplant surgeons are even using circaseptan cycles to improve transplant outcomes.[48]

All this begs the question: is there an internal seven-day cycle or has our "arbitrary" seven-day calendar imposed some discernible change in our physiology?[‡] I am sure you could have guessed that Mondays would be more stressful than Sundays and therefore account for more deaths, but this wouldn't explain why some plants and animals follow a circaseptan rhythm or why heart rate and both systolic and diastolic blood pressure in a study of individuals in a permanent vegetative state due to brain injury followed a strong circaseptan rhythm.[49]

---

† Circaseptan rhythm is considered one of many infradian rhythms that are defined as being longer than the normal circadian rhythm, such as weekly, bi-monthly, monthly, annually, etc. Ultradian rhythms are any cycles shorter than the circadian rhythm, like heart rate, pulsatile hormone release, etc.

‡ After the French Revolution, France instituted a ten-day week in an attempt to "decimalize" and remove religious influence from the culture. Allowing only one official rest day in ten was a bad idea, and they abandoned the French Revolutionary Calendar, as it was called, in 1805 after twelve years.

At this point we have yet to discover what I think we will find out in the future, that along with the highly controlled clock mechanism that drives the circadian rhythm, there is a set of mechanisms that keeps a steady seven-day cycle. But what is the zeitgeber, the external cue that helps to keep this cycle entrained? Some have suggested that solar or geomagnetic rhythms coincide with human circaseptan rhythms.[50] We just don't know yet. Until we find out, it appears that following a weekly pattern of work and rest, which happens to be engraved even upon the Supreme Court of the United States, is pretty good advice.

Ceasing labor for longer periods of time (a week or so) was also common in historical and traditional settings, often associated with post-harvest celebrations that would involve the whole community. These events were often holy days or days of thanksgiving that reinforced the bonds within the local community. Personal and small group retreats or pilgrimages were also part of human history throughout the past few millennia, when individuals spent various amounts of time away from their day-to-day tasks to pursue a spiritual/personal goal or adventure. Like our modern-day sabbatical, the individual often returned to their normal life with renewed vigor and purpose.

The concept of a personal "vacation" is a relatively recent invention, developed in the last two centuries. Prior to that time, *vacating* one's responsibilities for pleasure alone in a mostly rural and agrarian setting was a luxury only the wealthy could afford. In early America, groups like the Puritans frowned upon breaks from work for reasons other than weekly observance of the Sabbath. As labor changes occurred over the past few centuries, when individuals routinely began to labor for other people, however, the concept of a break from work took root amongst the middle and working classes.[51] Today, vacation time or holidays, as they are called in Europe, is an important part of keeping us healthy and stress-free.

Studies repeatedly support the health benefits of vacation time and the detriment to those who don't take enough time to get away. A study of 1500 rural women from Wisconsin found the odds of depression to be high in those who only took vacations once every two years compared to those who took vacations twice or more per year; further, their marital satisfaction also decreased with lower frequency of vacations.[52]

Frequent annual vacations even have a direct, inverse effect on mortality. Men with high risk for CHD who take more vacation time have a lower risk of mortality.[53,54] So if your life depends on taking a vacation, it is important to know that some vacations are more helpful than others. Even this has been studied.

What is the secret of an effective vacation, one that really provides the stress relief and rest that create these health benefits? What researchers have discovered isn't that big of a surprise. First, vacations don't necessarily need to be long (three days is sufficient) in order to give you a benefit as long as they have some important ingredients.[54] In fact, just planning a vacation will bring you the joy of anticipation for up to ten days prior to the vacation itself, measurably affecting mood and even physical complaints.[55] While on vacation, having enough time for yourself and your personal needs is also essential, as is the level of relaxation and freedom from obligation. Those who simply take time away without removing their obligations have much lower vacation benefits. Those who work while on vacation, well, they only vacate physically and gain very little benefit from the time away. Vacations including physical activity, good quality of sleep (not just quantity), and making new acquaintances are all positively associated with a feeling of recuperation.[54] Avoiding negative incidents and passive activities while on vacation also contributes to the positive effect of getting away.[56] Try to avoid non-work hassles such as conflicts within family or traffic as this will negatively impact you as well.[57] Finally, planning ahead to manage work tasks to avoid overload upon returning home is essential to make those great effects last as long as possible—until your next getaway.[57]

Humans are inextricably linked to the world around us. Whether we know it or not, modern technology cannot insulate us from our need to stay in time with all the natural rhythms around us. Our health, our sanity, and our life depend upon it.

CHAPTER 12

The Environmental Interface

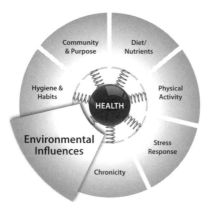

"Everybody needs beauty as well as bread,
places to play in and pray in, where nature may
heal and give strength to body and soul."

—John Muir (1838–1914)

WE HAVE ALREADY CATALOGUED dozens of lifestyle signals that have been altered by, added to, or removed from our human experience over the past few centuries. In this chapter, we will outline a number of these signals that can be generally grouped together as environmental interfaces—that is, signals that come from outside our body with or without our choice. Some of these environmental influences are quite damaging to our health and should be minimized or avoided, while others are influences that we should be encouraging. Each of these principles could easily be a chapter on its own, but we don't need to go into that much detail to allow you to see the signals provided by these environmental interfaces and what you can do about them. Since we always think of environmental influences as bad, we will begin with a familiar signal and show how environmental signals might be helpful.

Principle #1: Sunlight is more than a timekeeper for circadian rhythm—get a dose of sun on your skin for all its health benefits, but be careful not to overdo it.

In the last chapter, we talked quite a bit about sunlight being a strong signal for maintaining our circadian rhythm, but the "zeitgeber effect" of sunlight is based mostly upon the *timing* of the sunlight (sunrise, sunset, day length), which appears to be somewhat reproducible with experimental lights in a laboratory. Here we are not just talking about the timing of the light itself but about having direct access to sunlight on our skin. This will no doubt be controversial to some since we are more often reminded of the potential harm that can be induced by sunlight (i.e. skin cancer) than its many benefits.[†] So which benefits are we talking about?

Unless you have been under a rock for a while, you should be aware that the interest and appreciation for the sun-induced vitamin D has exploded throughout the world. Once thought of as a minor fat-soluble vitamin only needed to keep bones and teeth strong, vitamin D is now considered a vital substance that helps regulate a wide range of biological functions.[1] In some ways, vitamin D is not a vitamin at all. Unlike most other vitamins, we can produce our own vitamin D with adequate access to sunlight, and the active form of vitamin D acts more like a hormone than a traditional vitamin (see Sidebar on page 225).

So in a very real sense, ultraviolet light from the sun is capable of sending hormonal and genomic signals throughout your body using vitamin D as the messenger, unless, of course, you routinely avoid the sun in the summer months or cover yourself with clothing or sunscreen

---

[†] The recommendations of sun exposure in this book will differ from the position of many dermatologists. It is up to you and your clinician to determine the risk/reward of any therapy— even if it is lifestyle therapy. It is my view that the skin is designed to handle modest levels of sunlight (enough to slowly build up a tan, not burn the skin) when antioxidant levels in the skin are adequate.

that constantly blocks your skin's access to the sun. To give you some perspective: Twenty minutes of full torso access to sunlight will provide in the neighborhood of 2000 international units (IUs) of vitamin D, while one cup of fortified milk will provide only about 100 IUs. Using sunscreen of just SPF 8 blocks 95% of the skin's ability to make vitamin D_3, and anything more potent will block virtually all vitamin D synthesis. Here is where the controversy comes in: should we be recommending more access to sunlight (and less sunscreen) to combat vitamin D deficiency or vitamin D supplements instead?

According to many of the most prominent researchers on this topic, vitamin D deficiency is one of the most prevalent medical concerns on the planet and certainly the most prevalent in the U.S.[2,3] Currently, there is a debate about what blood levels of vitamin D constitute optimal levels and what should be viewed as insufficient or deficient levels. In 2010, the Institute of Medicine (IOM) increased the dietary recommendation of vitamin D by double or triple, depending on which age group you look at.[4] Even so, many believe the IOM's new recommendations are too conservative and, if followed, would still leave most Americans below the optimal serum vitamin D levels.†

The point here is not to review all the benefits of vitamin D; that would require another book of the same size as this. Instead, I hope to point out that just a few decades ago, our knowledge of this one "simple" vitamin as a signaling hormone was minimal. Today it is hard to go even a few months without seeing some important update about the latest findings on vitamin D. What appears as a deceivingly simple signal, in this case sunlight on the skin, turns out to be a trigger for a network of signals regulating almost every facet of our biology.

As you might remember from chapter 7, I listed vitamin D supplementation as an augmentation therapy. In this case, we should explain that a little more. Access to sunlight is the preferable (and natural) way to gain vitamin D, but access to sunlight may not be possible for some people or for all people all of the time. During most of the time between

---

† We have written a paper, "Target Serum Levels and Optimal Dosing of Vitamin D. A Response to the IOM Report," for clinicians that reviews the 2010 IOM report and argues for more appropriate blood level targets and supplemental vitamin D dosing. You can find it on our website, www.pointinstitute.org.

Vitamin D Deficiency

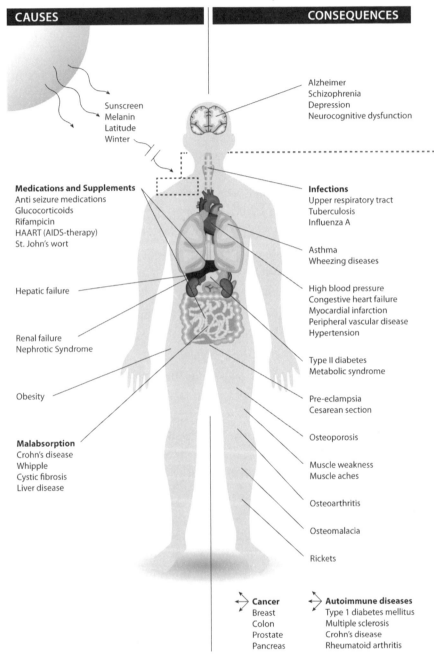

CAUSES

CONSEQUENCES

Sunscreen
Melanin
Latitude
Winter

Alzheimer
Schizophrenia
Depression
Neurocognitive dysfunction

Medications and Supplements
Anti seizure medications
Glucocorticoids
Rifampicin
HAART (AIDS-therapy)
St. John's wort

Infections
Upper respiratory tract
Tuberculosis
Influenza A

Asthma
Wheezing diseases

Hepatic failure

High blood pressure
Congestive heart failure
Myocardial infarction
Peripheral vascular disease
Hypertension

Renal failure
Nephrotic Syndrome

Type II diabetes
Metabolic syndrome

Pre-eclampsia
Cesarean section

Obesity

Osteoporosis

Malabsorption
Crohn's disease
Whipple
Cystic fibrosis
Liver disease

Muscle weakness
Muscle aches

Osteoarthritis

Osteomalacia

Rickets

Cancer
Breast
Colon
Prostate
Pancreas

Autoimmune diseases
Type 1 diabetes mellitus
Multiple sclerosis
Crohn's disease
Rheumatoid arthritis

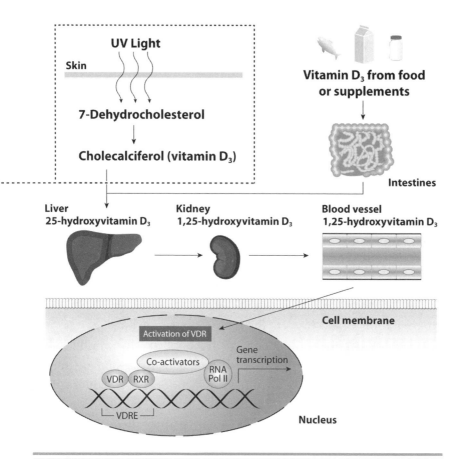

How We Produce Vitamin D

Our skin produces a molecule, derived from cholesterol, called 7-dehydrocholesterol. When ultraviolet light hits our skin, this molecule can be converted into cholecalciferol (vitamin D_3). Vitamin D_3 can also come as a preformed vitamin in our diet or through supplementation. Vitamin D_3 is still "inactive" at this point and must be converted to its active form by enzymes in the liver (to 25-hydroxyvitamin D_3 or 25(OH)D) and later the kidney (to 1,25-dihydroxyvitamin D_3 or 1,25(OH)$_2$D). The active form of vitamin D is able to enter the cell where it encounters the vitamin D receptor (VDR), and together they migrate into the nucleus to activate gene transcription (this is similar to cortisol signaling—see chapter 6). Thus, vitamin D is a potent regulator of many biological functions in a wide variety of cells.

late fall and early spring, those of us living in the northern hemisphere (especially in Wisconsin) have very little ability to make our own sun-induced vitamin D. Even if we chose to expose most of our body to the sun during these months, the distance and angle of the sunlight would not permit much vitamin D synthesis. Thankfully, vitamin D is fat-soluble and can be stored within the body, a handy design for those of us living in the north. High amounts of sunlight in the summer months produce elevated levels of vitamin D for storage in the winter months. Unfortunately, many people don't get enough sun exposure at any time during the year, diminishing their body's reserve of vitamin D. Today, we can augment this with vitamin D supplements, something I recommend highly.

How about sunscreen? My rule of thumb is to allow both adults and children to expose themselves to the sun for at least twenty to thirty minutes before putting on any sunscreen. This allows for the production of vitamin D and triggers the tanning response but then restricts additional UV irradiation after sunscreen is applied. My position is that we simply do not know what other beneficial signals sunlight might have in addition to those we have already mentioned. Prudent, regular, and careful exposure to the sun is part of a healthy lifestyle. Measuring vitamin D levels is a way to know if you are getting adequate sunlight. Avoid situations in which you are likely to sunburn. Supplementing with vitamin D may be an important way to augment the lack of sun exposure, but it is unlikely to be a substitute for all the beneficial signals that safe sun exposure is designed to elicit.

Principle #2: Toxic compounds are everywhere, and many are powerful signaling agents at very low doses. Be aware of the toxins around you, and maintain your detoxification capacity.

When we think of negative environmental influences on our health, usually the first things we think of are toxins. In our modern world, they are everywhere: in our air, water, food, clothing, prescription medication, cosmetics, detergents, building supplies, toys, and virtually everything else. In the U.S alone, there are over 80,000 synthetic chemicals in widespread use, with hundreds more being introduced weekly. While toxicity studies are required before new chemicals are widely used in the U.S., these studies cannot predict how each person might respond or how these compounds influence the toxicity of the thousands of other chemicals already in our environment. For most of the known chemicals in our environment, there is a lack of safety information, and the effect on health of multiple substances when used simultaneously is simply unknown. According to the Agency for Toxic Substances and Disease Registry (ATSDR), when just fifteen different combinations of toxic substances were tested, 41% were predicted to have additive effects, 20% to have synergistic effects, and for 24%, the minimum amount of information was lacking to form a conclusion. This lack of information is alarming since many of these compounds can affect us at very low doses, often at parts per billion (ppb).

Two related fields of study are beginning to help us discover the role toxins play in human health and disease, both owing to the emerging sciences of genetics and genomics. The first is the science known as toxicogenetics, which describes how the genetic differences between certain individuals allow for varying susceptibility to different toxins. Since there are hundreds of different enzymes involved in our detoxification pathways, some of us carry gene variants (polymorphisms) that allow us to more efficiently convert and remove toxins from our bodies than others. Those individuals with slower detoxification pathways will show signs of toxicity at much lower doses than those with normal detoxification capacity.

The second field of study that has emerged is based on how our body responds to toxins as a consequence of both immediate and lifetime exposures. In essence, which genes, proteins, and metabolites are altered under the influence of various toxins? The term toxicogenomics is used to describe these effects. Just as nutrigenomics tells us what genes are activated or repressed when we consume quercetin, so toxicogenomic studies tell us what genes are activated or repressed when our cells are exposed to a particular toxin, something like DDT. Another related term, the "exposome," has emerged to describe the total lifetime *exposure* to environmental agents that effect genomics (the mixed term for this is "exposomics").[5,6] The reason this is so important, and why so many new terms need to be created, is that the impact of toxins is both cumulative (over time) and synergistic (between different substances), requiring the overlapping of numerous disciplines. High doses of some toxins over a very short period of time may have one type of negative outcome, while smaller doses over a long period of time may have quite a different set of negative outcomes. Likewise, small doses of a particular toxin in a person with a strong detoxification capacity may have no discernible negative outcome at all, while the same or even lower dose in another person might lead to a wide range of abnormalities that often go unexplained.

There is a wealth of information about the negative health consequences of a number of specific toxins. Our principle here is to help you become aware of the toxins that may be around you and encourage you to avoid those which are likely to harm you. The following is a brief overview of some of the common toxins with wide-ranging health concerns—this is by no means a comprehensive review of the topic.[†]

Bisphenol-A (BPA)

We start with Bisphenol-A (BPA), not necessarily because it is the most harmful compound, but because of the attention it has received in the past few years. BPA is a widespread plasticizer found in polycarbonate bottles (such as baby bottles and water bottles), thermal paper, food cans, and a variety of other common, everyday products. In the past, infants and children were the most highly exposed to BPA, and this compound has been found at unsafe levels in maternal and umbilical cord blood, placental tissue, amniotic fluid, urine, and other bodily tissues. The international attention placed upon BPA lately has led to many changes in the manufacturing of certain items, especially those available for infants and children. It is quite common now to see "BPA-free" products being advertised.

As a toxin, BPA is classified as an endocrine disruptor, primarily affecting estrogen signaling. This disruption of hormone signaling is thought to affect reproduction as well as a number of other hormone-related processes, even changes to adipocytes, which may promote

---

[†] There is an excellent online resource from the Collaborative on Health and the Environment containing a searchable database that summarizes links between chemical contaminants and approximately 180 human diseases or conditions. You can search the database by either a condition or a toxin you may be concerned about. The website is http://www.healthandenvironment.org/tddb.

obesity.[7,8] BPA, along with many other toxins, is often considered to be "obesogenic" because of its ability to increase fat production.† Linking exposure to BPA (usually determined by urinary output of BPA metabolites) and specific outcomes is controversial since exposure limits are debated and there are many confounding factors.[9] Epidemiological studies (mostly cross-sectional), however, have clearly shown links between BPA exposure and increased risks for hypertension, diabetes, and obesity, as well as a number of non-cardiometabolic outcomes.[10–13] What is more alarming is the gathering research showing the epigenetic effects of BPA exposure in certain cells and tissues. Since we know that these effects can alter genetic expression, and even cell differentiation and development if exposure is early enough, epigenetic and toxicogenomic studies (animal and human cell culture studies) are leading the way to hint at how these compounds cause long-term human disease outcomes.[14,15] There is a silver lining in some of this research, however. Recall the Agouti mouse model we discussed earlier as the premier model for epigenetic influence through DNA methylation. It turns out that in this mouse model, BPA will also induce hypomethylation, a phenomenon that is negated when the mouse is fed methyl-donors such as folate or genistein (from soy).[16] So while it is true that avoidance of toxins is still the key to protecting ourselves and our future offspring, we may be able to decrease or even eliminate our susceptibility for these toxins by maintaining other healthy lifestyle inputs, especially the diet.

Phthalates

Phthalates are compounds used in the production of most plastics to impart flexibility and resilience. They are also found in adhesives, glues, detergents, flooring, shower curtains, personal care products (shampoos, cosmetics, etc.), plastic bags, paints, pharmaceuticals, and building materials. Since they are not chemically bound to the plastics to which they are added, they are easily released into the environment and reach especially high levels in indoor air, where they are thought to contribute to lung-related disorders.[17]

---

† Since most toxic compounds are fat-soluble, it seems logical that the body would have a way to protect itself by storing toxins in fatty tissues and diluting the toxin by further increasing fat mass—recalling the old adage "The solution to pollution is dilution." This is another reason I view fat mass as the terminal buffering system of the body.

Like BPA, phthalates are known endocrine disruptors, and high doses have been shown to alter hormone levels and lead to birth defects, especially in the development of the male reproductive system.[18] In two national cross-sectional studies of men in the U.S., an increased concentration of phthalate metabolites was significantly correlated with insulin resistance and abnormal obesity that the authors suggested may be mediated through toxin-induced testosterone depletion.[19] In elderly women, specific phthalate metabolites have been recently linked to increased abdominal fat gain over just a two-year period.[20] Currently, few epigenetic and toxicogenomic studies have been conducted using phthalates, although it is likely that these mechanisms are at least partly responsible for the outcomes related to phthalate exposure.

Dioxins

Dioxins refer to one specific compound (dioxin- 2,3,7,8-tetrachlorodibenzo para dioxin (TCDD)) and related dioxin-like compounds. Dioxins are generally byproducts of industrial processes and are commonly used in the paper bleaching process, chemical and pesticide manufacturing, and combustion activities (incineration of waste, burning of trash, etc.). According to the WHO, "*although formation of dioxins is local, environmental distribution is global. Dioxins are found throughout the world in the environment. The highest levels of these compounds are found in some soils, sediments and food, especially dairy products, meat, fish and shellfish. Very low levels are found in plants, water and air.*"[21] As far back as 1994, the U.S. EPA reported that dioxins at very low levels are a probable carcinogen but also reported that their non-cancer causing effects (reproductive, sexual development, and immune system issues) may pose an even greater threat to human health. Epidemiological studies have shown that exposure to high levels of dioxins leads to an increased risk of tumors at all sites.

Dioxins are known to bind to a receptor known as the Aryl hydrocarbon receptor (AhR), which acts to alter the genetic expression of numerous genes, including those expressing certain detoxification enzymes. The alteration of these genes, and their subsequent proteins, can increase the level of toxic intermediates and is thought to be the main signaling pathway in dioxin-induced toxicity.[22] In animal models, the phytonutrient resveratrol has been shown to be able to diminish dioxin's toxic effects.[23] Likewise, the cruciferous compounds indole-3-carbonole (I3C) and diindolylmethane (DIM) have modulating effects, which differ based on timing and dose, on the AhR-dependent response.[24]

Toxic Metals

Certain metals/minerals, often called "heavy metals" because of their molecular weight, are known to be toxic to humans. The most common of these are mercury, lead, cadmium, arsenic, and aluminum. These metals are commonly found in cookware, dental fillings, antiperspirants, batteries, foods, fertilizers, water, and tobacco smoke. Acute poisoning from high doses of heavy metals is well documented and won't be discussed here. Instead, we will focus on the fact that chronic environmental exposures can cause heavy metals to accumulate in our tissues, which has been linked to the increased risk of various chronic diseases. The effects of metal compounds on human health have been called "metallomics."

Mercury (Hg): Chronic exposure to mercury, arguably the most persistently harmful heavy metal in our environment, has been associated with numerous health consequences. The U.S. population is primarily exposed to mercury in the form of methyl-mercury by consuming fish and seafood (which act as terminal bio-accumulators from the aquatic food chain). The guideline cautioning against overconsumption of fish, including canned tuna, especially for pregnant women and children, is designed to limit mercury ingestion during fetal and early child development. Other common sources of mercury are drugs for the eye, ear, nose, throat, and skin; bleaching creams; preservatives in cosmetics, toothpastes, lens solutions, vaccines, allergy tests, and immunotherapy solutions; antiseptics, disinfectants, and contraceptives; fungicides and herbicides; and dental fillings and thermometers. While somewhat controversial, the overwhelming preponderance of the evidence favors acceptance that mercury exposure, from multiple sources, is capable of causing some forms of autism.[25]

Several studies have shown a correlation between heart disease and chronic mercury exposure.[26] One case-control study of 684 men found a significant association between mercury levels (15% increased mercury toenail content) and first-time heart attack in men compared to controls.[27] A study of European mercury miners found a significant relationship between mercury exposure and total mortality, hypertension, heart disease, renal disease, and stroke.[28] Mercury's mechanisms of toxicity are not well understood but appear to be based on four main processes that lead to genotoxicity: the generation of free radicals and oxidative stress, action on microtubules (part of the structural network within the cell), influence on DNA repair mechanisms, and direct interaction with DNA molecules.[29] Mercury, in particular, depletes certain tissues of the important antioxidant glutathione because it binds so tightly to other thiol groups. Substances that increase glutathione levels have been shown to reduce the toxic effects of mercury in some models,[†] including N-acetyl cysteine, alpha-lipoic acid, lycopene, proanthocyanins, polyphenols from tea, quercetin, and even garlic.[30-36] The minerals zinc and selenium have also been shown to inhibit some of the toxic effects of mercury.[37]

Lead (Pb): The harmful effects of lead have been well-known and documented for years. Even in antiquity, the mining and use of lead were known to cause toxicity. Today, while we have ceased using lead in gasoline and paint here in the U.S., according to the CDC there are still approximately 24 million housing units (most built prior to 1978) with deteriorated lead paint and elevated levels of lead-contaminated house dust.[38] Likewise, environmental air, water, and especially soil lead levels allow certain crops to concentrate lead levels (even organic products). Lead exposure is known to affect neuronal development and the function of a variety of organ systems, including the cardiovascular, renal, and reproductive systems.

The toxic mechanism of lead is not completely understood. Like mercury, lead also is a strong oxidant that depletes cell antioxidants, especially thiols like glutathione. Lead also interferes with calcium function and reduces nitric oxide signaling (which is important for

---

† Thiol or sulfhydryl groups are found on proteins, amino acids, and cellular metabolites. Some of the substances listed here are thought to bind or chelate mercury due to mercury's affinity for these compounds, in addition to increasing glutathione levels directly.

cardiovascular function).[39,40] You might suspect that if the depletion of antioxidants is part of the "signals" of lead toxicity, then antioxidants might be able to diminish the negative effects of lead toxicity, and it appears there is some evidence to suggest this might be so.[41,42] Chelating agents, however, are the method of choice for therapeutic reduction of body lead levels.

Other Toxic Metals: There are a few other toxic metals you might want to keep in mind such as arsenic (As), cadmium (Cd), and aluminum (Al). Arsenic is a particularly toxic metal still found in drinking water in some locations in the U.S. Arsenic can also be found in older "green-treated" lumber. Common sources of cadmium in the U.S. include fossil fuel combustion, phosphate fertilizers, municipal solid waste incineration, and iron, steel, and cement production. Smoking, however, is the most important single source of cadmium exposure in the general population. While arsenic effectively inhibits cells from producing ATP, the energy molecule in the cell, cadmium exerts its toxic effect by binding to the endoplasmic reticulum and mimicking estrogen.[43,44] Chronic exposure to arsenic manifests in many ways, mostly through the production of reactive oxygen species (free radicals), which places a burden on the antioxidant network. Links to metabolic diseases (especially insulin resistance and type 2 diabetes) as well as some cancers are the most frequently cited with chronic low-dose arsenic exposure.[45–47]

The issue of aluminum is a bit more complex. Research appears to clearly link aluminum neurotoxicity with the risk for Alzheimer's disease.[48] A debate exists about the cause-effect relationship between aluminum exposure and Alzheimer's disease progression. Some studies, such as the PAQUID cohort,[49] identify aluminum exposure as a risk factor for Alzheimer's disease, and cell culture studies have found that neuritic plaques contain increased levels of aluminum.[49,50] Other studies have shown increased population risks for Alzheimer's disease with elevated aluminum concentrations in public drinking water supplies.[51] Although the data is incomplete, an increasing number of researchers have expressed concern that aluminum found in certain deodorants may increase the risk of breast cancer and have implicated aluminum as a factor in Alzheimer's disease.[52,53] In addition, higher levels of aluminum have been found in the urine of multiple sclerosis (MS) patients, with even higher levels found in the relapsing-remitting form of MS.

Pesticides

Pesticides are not only sprayed onto our food (especially fruits and vegetables) but seep into our soil and groundwater, and can end up in our drinking water and the air. Pesticides (such as chlorinated pesticides) have been found in the breast milk of women from all over the globe.[54,55] Furthermore, chlorinated pesticide residues (such as DDT, DDE, DDD, aldrin, dieldrin, heptachlor, heptachlor epoxide, and PCBs) have been detected in the adipose tissue from residents living in the U.S., Europe, Israel, Africa, and even Greenland.[56-60] Various studies have documented the presence of these pesticides in maternal umbilical cord blood,[61-64] and chronic exposure to pesticides has been shown to be associated with numerous adverse health effects, from simple irritation of the skin and eyes[65-67] to hormonal disruption,[68,69] neurotox-

Figure 12.2. **Contaminants in Conventionally Grown Fruits and Vegetables**

Dirty Dozen *Buy These Organic*		Clean 15 *Lowest in Pesticides*	
WORST	1 Apples	BEST	1 Onions
	2 Celery		2 Corn
	3 Strawberries		3 Pineapples
	4 Peaches		4 Avocado
	5 Spinach		5 Asparagus
	6 Nectarines		6 Sweet Peas
	7 Grapes		7 Mangos
	8 Sweet Bell Peppers		8 Eggplant
	9 Potatoes		9 Cantaloupe
	10 Blueberries		10 Kiwi
	11 Lettuce		11 Cabbage
	12 Kale / Collard Greens		12 Watermelon
			13 Sweet Potatoes
			14 Grapefruit
			15 Mushrooms

icity,[70,71] and carcinogenic activity.[72-74] Exposure during pregnancy to endocrine-disrupting chemicals such as polycyclic aromatic hydrocarbons has been found to increase the risk of childhood obesity.[75] A 2007 systematic review found that most studies on non-Hodgkin lymphoma and leukemia had positive associations with pesticide exposure,[76] and strong evidence also exists for other negative outcomes from pesticide exposure including birth defects,[77,78] fetal death,[79] and neurodevelopmental disorders.[80]

The use of pesticides and herbicides on "healthy" fruits and vegetables has led many to consider using organically-grown produce, a trend that is expanding rapidly in the U.S.[†] In order to maximize the cost and value of organically-grown produce, focus your organic purchases on those fruits and vegetables known to have the highest amounts of added chemicals in the conventional growing environment (See the "Dirty Dozen" chart).

Principle #3: Hidden allergies and sensitivities can create a chronic health burden. Know and avoid the things to which you are allergic and sensitive.

An allergic reaction is a highly coordinated immune system response to substances that are for the most part harmless. The immune reaction, however, is not harmless and triggers a potent inflammatory response. If you are constantly exposing yourself to substances that are triggering these immune and inflammatory signals, you are likely creating or exacerbating symptoms that have become part of your "normal" life. Some of these symptoms you recognize, while others are less obvious. Of course, when these allergic reactions are accompanied by the itching and sneezing we traditionally associate with seasonal airborne or contact allergies, it is easy to pinpoint our allergic vulnerabilities. Many allergens, especially food allergens, will present much more subtly, perhaps for some as a dull headache or joint pain, or maybe a scratchy throat or sinus drainage; for others as lethargy; and for others GI complaints. The allergic response might be immediate, making

---

† While there is an ongoing debate about whether organically-grown produce has higher levels of vitamins, minerals, or phytonutrients, there is little debate about the fact that organically-grown produce contains fewer toxic herbicides, pesticides, and fungicides.

it easier to connect the symptoms with the substance, but very often it takes hours or even days for the symptoms to appear, making the connection difficult to trace.

In some cases, you might be consuming reactive substances so often that the symptoms are always present—you've just never related them to your diet or daily routine. In order to discover the possible connection between hidden food allergies and symptoms you might be experiencing, you have basically two options: have a clinician perform tests to identify your allergic sensitivities, or eliminate all potentially reactive foods, then reintroduce each substance one at a time. The second option, in my opinion, is better because it allows the body to define a wider array of symptoms than what might be detected using skin or blood tests. Nevertheless, the key is eliminating the substance long enough to allow the immune reaction to subside so that reintroduction can spark a noticeable response. One of the easiest ways to do this is to eliminate all potentially reactive foods at the same time (elimination diet). For most this might mean starting with the eight common food allergens required for labeling: wheat, milk, eggs, fish, shellfish, peanuts, tree nuts, and soy. You may also want to consider eliminating corn, rye, barley, and plants in the nightshade family, such as potatoes, tomatoes, eggplant, and peppers, as these can be problematic as well. You must eliminate these from your diet for at least two weeks to notice a "response" when reintroducing them. When reintroducing each food category, record any symptoms you feel for at least two to three days before reintroducing the next food category. If you can discover one or more hidden food allergens or food sensitivities that might be driving chronic inflammation and secondary symptoms, you can help your body immensely by removing the food from your diet.† The same is true of common household products and personal care items: have you

---

† Performing an elimination diet along with a protocol to improve detoxification capacity is being recommended by a number of doctors who understand the complexity of the role of both the liver and GI in managing our immune system response. A protocol like this is recommended on an annual or semi-annual basis by many of these clinicians.

ever stopped to think about whether you have adverse reactions to your shampoo, deodorant, cosmetics, soaps, detergents, etc.?

Principle #4: Electromagnetic fields are everywhere; be aware of your exposure, and consider ways to reduce their negative impact.

Unless you live "off the grid," electromagnetic fields (EMFs) are all around you. From electric power lines to cell phones, the flow of electricity through an object creates a small or large field of electromagnetic influence upon the objects around it. There is no doubt that humans respond to EMFs ; the question is whether exposure to human-made EMFs has negative health consequences. In the past few decades, growing numbers of studies have begun to explore the effects of EMFs on our health, and it appears there is some concern and quite a bit of controversy. Without getting bogged down in the nuances and debates, it is clear that humans are being exposed to more electromagnetic and radio fields than ever before in history, and the proximity and frequency of our contact with these energy fields continues to grow. For instance, we can sleep all night under an electric blanket with our head just inches from our alarm clock (in fact, some of our homes or apartments are located near power lines). When we wake, we might plop our laptop onto our lap; turn on the TV, the lights, and the coffeemaker; and check our voicemails with our cell phone up against our ear. A person living just 150 years ago would have no opportunity to expose their body to such concentrated EMFs.

Some epidemiological studies suggest that EMFs have been related to skin, muscular, and GI disturbances; fatigue; headaches; and concentration problems in people with electromagnetic hypersensitivity (EHS).[81] Numerous other studies related to EMFs suggest the increased risk of leukemia, brain tumors, genotoxic effects, neurology effects, neurodegenerative disease, immune dysregulation, allergic inflammatory response, breast cancer, miscarriage, and cardiovascular effects.[82] Since the data is currently difficult to interpret and controversial, we suggest what some call "prudent avoidance." This basically means that you keep your distance, when possible, from strong sources of EMFs (you can purchase a Gauss meter to determine the EMF exposure of various appliances). Focus on the places you spend the most time: your bedroom, your office or workplace, your favorite chair. Use hands-free options for your cell phone, and don't put your laptop directly on your lap. Until we know more about what sources, doses, and mechanisms of EMF-related concerns we need to avoid, being aware and prudently avoiding unnecessary exposure appears to be the best approach.

Principle #5: Get in direct contact with nature (with the earth and its beauty) as often as possible; create a buffer from modernity.

Why is it that we long to enjoy just sitting in the outdoors, perhaps beside a gently meandering brook or a quiet little lake, far beyond the noises of the city, where the only sounds are the breeze and the birds? Ask someone to describe "heaven" and they are more likely to describe some "earthly" scene like this than any other. No matter how fancy our gadgets become, they cannot replace the need to touch and see the natural beauty around us. Researchers have tried to define this in various ways, and, as you can imagine, it has been difficult to investigate.

While seemingly obvious, access to beautiful natural landscapes has been shown to improve both mental and physical outcomes, although these effects are sometimes difficult to measure.[83] Studies have confirmed that exposure to natural settings results in stress reduction, improved attention, and increased cognitive function after intense mental activity.[84] Green environments have been found to improve self-esteem and mood, an effect enhanced by increasing our proximity to water (perhaps the intrinsic value of waterfront property has its roots here).[84] Just viewing natural scenes reduces symptoms of ADHD, improves self-discipline, reduces aggression and crime, promotes better health in the elderly, and even delays the impact of Alzheimer's disease. Furthermore, it is known that hospital patients recover faster when facing trees, prison inmates are healthier when viewing landscapes, and citizens report more feelings of tranquility, peace, and relaxation when viewing savanna-like scenes.[85]

Exactly what is being triggered by viewing or experiencing an aesthetically beautiful landscape is difficult to determine, which is one of the reasons such studies are difficult to interpret and repeat. Regardless, our ability to appreciate natural beauty is an inalienable part of the human design that can only be generated when we get outdoors and experience the expanse of nature. Maybe for a few minutes (is there a park nearby?), a few hours, or even for weeks at a time, find a place you can go to get away and put yourself in a natural setting, preferably by water.

Another fairly recent area of investigation that I find interesting is related to our physical connectedness with the earth itself. Many have noted that in our sophisticated modern world we have virtually insulated ourselves from being in contact with the earth. Think about how often you touch the earth without something in between (your shoes, gloves, concrete, etc.); in fact, many of us spend much of our time not just insulated but separated from the earth by several layers of concrete and air (unless you work or live on the ground level with no basement below). In antiquity, humans lived, walked, slept, and sat directly on the earth nearly twenty-four hours a day. Some new research suggests that when we are connected directly to the earth, a certain electrical equilibrium is maintained between our bodies and the ground that promotes overall health.[86] In fact, some proponents recommend "earthing" or "grounding" in the form of regular barefoot contact with the earth and even placing specific wiring mechanisms to "ground" the bed you sleep on. It might surprise you, but sleeping on a "grounded" bed has been shown to change numerous physiological measurements in a positive manner. One study looking at circadian cortisol profiles in those grounded during sleep found measurable improvements in blood cortisol levels. Symptoms such as sleep dysfunction, pain, and stress were reduced or eliminated in almost all subjects, and these changes were most apparent in females.[87] Another study found that the continuous "earthing" of the body using a copper conductor decreased blood glucose in diabetic patients as well as modulating sodium, potassium, magnesium, albumin concentrations, transferrin, ferritin, and other blood proteins.[88]

With everything else we already know about the signals that drive our health, it is not too much of a stretch to think that regular contact with the earth may provide a very subtle signal that helps calibrate the electrical process of our physiology. You can decide whether the data is strong enough to suggest grounding your bed, but we at least recommend taking your shoes off in the outdoors as often as is practical, perhaps even creating a time to go barefoot on a regular basis.

Principle #6: Life has a soundtrack; be sure the sounds around you are making you healthy.

Nearly every culture from virtually every corner of the world uses music or sound (drum beats) to affect a broad sense of mood amongst a group of individuals; these sounds are often part of what distinguishes one culture from another. In fact, if you close your eyes through much of a modern movie, you could easily describe the type of scene being depicted just by the music the director uses to accompany the action. Music is a powerful tool, one that can be used for many outcomes; but would it surprise you that a person's blood pressure can be increased or decreased just by changing the type of music in a doctor's office? It's true.[89] It is now well known that both good noise and bad noise have a strong effect on our physiology and mood,† even changing our pain tolerance.[90]

According to some researchers, the greatest health benefits seem to be associated with listening to classical and meditative music, particularly Bach, Mozart, and Italian composers, not only increasing happiness but also reducing cardiovascular risk factors.[90] The opposite might also be the case; a recent report at the American Society of Hypertension (ASH) 2012 Scientific Sessions showed that blood pressure was lower when listening to a Mozart adagio but significantly higher while listening to the rock band Queen's "Bicycle Race." Of course, with the ease of downloading music at the click of a mouse, today we can create our own soundtrack for life. Sometimes our music creates our mood, other times our mood dictates our music. I have several playlists on my mp3 player (I am partial to bluegrass music) that I can choose depending on my mood, some upbeat, some slower, some vocal, some instrumental. I would like to think that most of the music stored in my mp3 player is promoting my health—how about yours?

---

† The biblical account of David's music being used to calm King Saul's spiritual and emotional mood is an ancient witness to the power of the effects of music on an individual.

Principle #7: Your body hosts trillions of good bacteria—your health depends on how well you guard this "environment."

This is a huge and important topic but one whose details are well beyond the scope of this book. As a principle to maintaining our health, however, understanding how we can sustain a healthy interface with the trillions of bacteria that exist on or in our bodies is vital. Likewise, our general ignorance of the benefits of good bacteria has led to a number of negative health consequences.

The most studied of the good bacteria exist in our gastrointestinal tract, an environment that is, technically, still outside the body. Within our GI tract are trillions of bacteria divided into 400–500 different subspecies. This microbiome, as it is called, helps us digest our food, produces important metabolic substrates and vitamins, protects us from harmful bacteria, detoxifies harmful substances, helps us maintain bowel regularity, and is very critical in maturing our immune system response. When the microbiome is disturbed in any way, we call this dysbiosis, and a wide range of symptoms can ensue.[91] The following are tips you can use to help be the best host possible:

- Limit your intake of antibiotics to only those that are absolutely necessary. Numerous antibiotics create a dysbiosis in the gut that gives an advantage to harmful bacteria and yeast organisms. This imbalance makes it very difficult to regain a proper environment for a healthy microbiome, often resulting in antibiotic-associated diarrhea (AAD) and infections by the bacterium *Clostridium difficile* (C. diff.).[92,93] This is especially damaging when chronic use of antibiotics occurs during childhood and adolescence when the microbiome superstructure (biofilm) is being formed.

- Be careful not to overdo antibiotic hand soaps and antiseptic gels. As we will mention in chapter 13, our fear of germs has led to overaggressive use of antibiotics in drugs, in hand soaps, and even in raising animals. Good old soap and hot water are adequate for nearly all applications. Save the hand gel for when you have no soap and water available or are in particular environments where contamination is likely.

- Don't fear getting dirty. Researchers now believe that our lack of contact with dirt (clean dirt!), along with all the soil bacterial organisms, is preventing us from creating a balanced gut micro-biome, which has resulted in poor immune maturation. This hygiene hypothesis is thought to contribute to the higher prevalence of allergies and autoimmune diseases in our hyper-clean environment.[94]

- Use probiotics to help maintain a healthy gut microbial environment. Some of the most popular dietary supplements in the world today are probiotics—healthy microbial organisms that are delivered in the form of functional foods (yogurt), capsules, tablets, or pouches. Doses ranging from a few billion to over a trillion have been studied for a wide range of clinical conditions with positive outcomes. While there are numerous strains or species of probiotics, I usually recommend a comprehensive blend of Lactobacillus and Bifidobacterium strains. The use of probiotics is now common to prevent and treat AAD (I recommend everyone use probiotics if they have to take an antibiotic) as well as a host of other specific gastrointestinal complaints.[95–97]

While you may not be able to control all the input signals from the environment around you, there are many ways that you can influence your ability to maximize the beneficial signals and decrease the detrimental signals. Think about your weekly routine in light of the principles discussed in this chapter. How can you adjust your routine to shift the interface with these inputs to improve the healthy signals your body will receive next week?

CHAPTER 13

Habits that Haunt, Habits that Heal

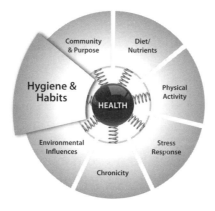

"Bad habits are easier to abandon today than tomorrow."
—Yiddish Proverb

THROUGHOUT THIS BOOK, WE have listed many things that have changed over the past few centuries that have harmed our health, both as individuals and as populations. However, improvements in hygiene practices are a silver lining amongst those many negative influences. Especially related to the limitation of communicable and contagious diseases, improved hygiene practices of waste disposal, food and beverage preparation and storage, and medical practices are largely responsible for reducing the outbreak of many illnesses of previous generations.[†]

[†] There are still many areas of the world where, for economic or other reasons, modern hygiene practices are yet to be fully implemented. In these areas, many of these diseases still exist and, due to the ease of world travel, sometimes still affect Western nations.

Many of these practices are mandated by governmental agencies and inspected by auditors to ensure proper compliance. Personal hygiene practices are still needed in order for us to fully gain the benefit of these advancements; likely, we were taught many of these things by our mothers, the domestic version of the government auditor.

Hygiene is an old medical concept related to both personal and professional care practices. In medical and domestic settings, hygiene practices are used to prevent and reduce the incidence and spread of disease. Often tied together with cleanliness, hygiene really refers to practices that prevent the spread of disease-causing organisms. Along with the good habits of personal hygiene, we want to discuss some very specific habits that can negatively affect your health as well. Some of these are fairly well established, being a part of well-known government or medical public health intervention programs. We include them here and discuss them briefly because they can be profoundly important to improve the health of individuals. Since readers of this book are likely familiar with these topics already, we won't attempt to nag.

Principle #1: Keep yourself and your surroundings free of filth, and don't forget about the organisms you cannot see.

Perhaps the most well-known practice of good hygiene is hand washing, especially after using the bathroom or before preparing food. Hand washing is even a symbolic sign of purity in many religions. It is hard to believe that in the fairly recent past clinicians would routinely move from patient to patient without washing their hands—today this would be grounds for a lawsuit. Each year, public health announcements remind us that we can become infected with respiratory illnesses such as influenza or the common cold if we don't wash our hands before touching our eyes, nose, or mouth; they also tell us about door knobs, keyboards, phones, and numerous other places that can harbor infectious agents.

Not satisfied to remove dirt alone, our zeal to kill off all potentially harmful organisms has gone pharmaceutical. In recent years, antibiotic soaps and hand sanitizers have become almost ubiquitous. This strategy, as logical as it may at first seem, has opened up a debate about the potential hazards of using antibacterial compounds so widely. In the U.S., one of the most commonly used chemical biocide agents in hygiene-related products is triclosan. A 2007 review found that soaps containing triclosan were no more effective than plain soaps at preventing the spread of infectious illness or reducing hand bacteria.[1] In fact, several studies have shown evidence that triclosan promotes cross-resistance to antibiotics among several bacterial species.[1] Bacterial resistance to antibiotics is becoming a major problem that continues to grow each year and is directly linked to the overuse of antibiotics in medicine, agriculture, and hygiene-related products. This obsession with a sterile environment and the consequences of poor immune system maturation are part of the "hygiene hypothesis" discussed in the previous chapter. Ever-increasing levels of excessive hygiene have even been linked to the increase in atopic diseases, such as allergies and asthma,[2-4] and cardiometabolic diseases.[5] Nevertheless, simple hand washing is still an important practice for reducing the transmission of infectious diseases in the community setting as well as in clinical settings.[1]

The same is true of washing one's clothes, bedding, furniture, and common household surfaces that routinely come in contact with our hands or food. As we mentioned previously, most of this is regulated in the public sphere but is sometimes woefully neglected in our homes. How often do you ensure the cutting surfaces of your kitchen are properly cleaned before placing food that will not later be cooked upon them? How often do you clean the TV remote after you stay home with the flu? We need to be diligent, just not fanatical, when it comes to cleanliness.

Principle #2: Maintaining good oral and dental hygiene is vital for your health.

When it comes to dental health, modernization over the past few centuries has two prevailing trends. The first involves a degeneration of dental health due to changes in diet and nutrition; the second is the improvement of technologies to counter the negative effects of the first. The classic text by Weston A. Price, DDS, *Nutrition and Physical Degeneration*, catalogs the dental health of primitive peoples prior to and after adopting Western lifestyles and foods. His discovery was simply that prior to Westernization, indigenous people had very well-developed facial and dental formation and were relatively free of dental caries, but after Western foods were introduced dental caries became quite high. Furthermore, the longer a society followed these Western dietary patterns, the more likely individuals were to suffer with facial and dental deformities. Today, since most of the world is consuming a Western-style diet, this dental burden must be combatted using modern methods of oral hygiene. This important augmentation to the foundations of good nutrition is critical for good oral health and for much more than merely dental-related issues.†

A recent survey by the American Heart Association (AHA) found that 25% of Americans admit they don't practice proper oral hygiene by brushing twice a day and flossing once a day.[6] Why, you ask, would the AHA care about proper oral hygiene; aren't they just concerned about cardiovascular issues? It should come as no surprise that maintaining good oral hygiene, including regular brushing and flossing and dental check-ups, is not just about keeping your teeth white and clean. The effects of neglecting good oral hygiene, such as gingivitis and gum disease, will impact many other aspects of health throughout the body. For instance, it has long been known that there is a direct link between periodontal disease and atherosclerosis; so those bacteria from our mouth may contribute to development of cardiovascular disease if we are not brushing and flossing regularly.[7] This is why the AHA cares about your teeth!

More than that, new research may have even linked certain oral bacteria with the development of obesity in humans. In one cross-sectional study of obese adolescents and normal-weight subjects, bacterial cells in subgingival biofilm were significantly associated with obesity.[8] Another study also found that the oral bacterial populations of overweight women were different than those of normal-weight women; one bacterium in particular, *Selenomonas noxia*, was identified in 98.4% of overweight women.[9] These are preliminary reports and small cross-sectional populations, but it is very interesting data nonetheless and mirrors current research that also suggests certain GI bacterial populations (gut microbiota) correlate with obesity.[10] Whether these two phenomena are linked is currently unknown, but both are thought to increase

---

† There is a wealth of information about the proper ways to prevent tooth decay and the means to "fix" the teeth if they have become infected. Our only general advice here would be to seek out solutions that do not add additional toxic burdens to the body.

inflammatory signaling, which is part of the obesity/metabolic disease mechanism. And just as with other areas of modern research, genomic influence of this oral microbiome is currently being researched to see what genetic and metabolic signaling is coming from this unique ecosystem we harbor in our mouth.[11,12]

Principle #3: Do we really need to say it? Smoking is a deadly habit and must be stopped if you are to become healthy.

The adverse health effects from cigarette smoking account for an estimated 443,000 deaths, or nearly one of every five deaths, each year in the U.S. More deaths are caused each year from tobacco use than human immunodeficiency virus (HIV), illegal drug use, alcohol use, motor vehicle injuries, suicides, and murders combined. Smoking causes an estimated 90% of all lung cancer deaths in men and 80% of all lung cancer deaths in women.[13] Of course, we can rehearse more statistics if you would like.

As a lifestyle intervention, smoking cessation programs, along with programs designed to curtail smoking initiation amongst young people, are responsible for saving countless lives and should be encouraged for any current smoker or vulnerable teen. Early prevention is key, as the recent surgeon general's report claims that 99% of current smokers began smoking before age 26.[14] While the rate of cigarette use has generally declined, the report still claimed that one in four high school seniors is a regular cigarette smoker.

Cigarette smoke is a toxic substance that carries with it a number of specific harmful signals, both as direct oxidant and damaging molecules and as triggers for changes in gene expression and epigenetic modification.[15–17] Unfortunately, one of those signals is in the form of the alkaloid nicotine, a highly addictive substance that makes it very difficult to stop smoking without significant withdrawal symptoms. At least in mice, nicotine creates epigenetic changes that increase the addictive power of cocaine, another highly addictive alkaloid.[18]

If you are reading this book and you are a current smoker, I implore you to seek out a competent smoking cessation program. Seeking to be healthy while refusing to give up cigarettes is a compromise you should not accept; it makes as much sense as attempting to save money on your heating bill by burning a $5 bill once per day. If you have a loved one who smokes or are making recommendations for others, helping them quit smoking is one of the greatest things you could do to improve their health (and their finances, and that awful smell on their clothes. …)

Principle #4: While some research suggests that low amounts can be part of a healthy lifestyle, the potential dangers of alcohol consumption require most individuals to avoid it altogether.

Alcohol consumption, especially in the U.S., is a complex and divisive topic. Approximately 79,000 deaths are attributable to excessive alcohol use each year in the U.S., making it the third leading lifestyle-related cause of death.[19] Since many of these deaths occur in young people, excessive alcohol use is responsible for 2.3 million years of potential life lost (YPLL) annually, which is about thirty years of potential life lost for each death.[19] When we add the social consequences of alcohol abuse to these statistics, the picture is quite sobering.

Complicating this topic is a number of studies that appear to show consumption of beverages containing moderate levels of alcohol can be part of a healthy lifestyle—even showing specific health benefits of both beer and red wine, for instance. The debate about whether the benefits come from the alcohol content or the related phytonutrients "extracted" during the making of these products is still quite vigorous. Reviews on the topic show that light to moderate amounts of polyphenol-rich beverages like wine or beer improve measurements of immunity in healthy adults as well as decrease total mortality, development of peripheral arterial disease, ischemic stroke, sudden cardiac death, heart attacks, angina, and even some cancers.[20–22] And, of course, red wine is notably part of the Mediterranean diet.

Ethanol is a strong antiseptic agent that inhibits the growth of bacteria and fungus. This property allowed fermented drinks, which naturally contained small amounts of ethanol, to be safely stored and used throughout most of recorded history.† Ethanol is also a strong signal to the body and considered to be a toxin at a fairly low threshold (which differs based

---

† Archeological evidence suggests that nearly every culture in antiquity had some form of fermented drink as part of their society. The Bible even records that Noah planted a vineyard amongst his post-flood activities, soon thereafter becoming drunk from the wine produced by his vineyard (Gen. 9:20–21).

upon the blood volume of the individual and their ethanol detoxification efficiency). We also know that alcohol modifies gene expression and creates epigenetic modifications that may be passed along to offspring from either parent.[23-25] All of these modifications appear to be harmful, rather than protective, for the outcome of the tissues or offspring.

It is for these reasons that we advise against alcohol consumption for optimal health. As modern techniques allow for the consumption of polyphenol-rich beverages that no longer require fermentation or added alcohol to prevent spoilage, we suggest using these non-alcoholic beverages instead. Since there is data suggesting moderate alcohol consumption is not, per se, detrimental to overall health (perhaps even benefiting some aspects), however, we would add that responsible alcohol consumption (if you choose to imbibe) should be strictly practiced prior to conception (by both potential parents) and during gestation to ensure limited influence on your child.

Principle #5: Stay sober and healthy; avoid the use of all illicit and addictive drugs.

This principle is pretty obvious, so we won't spend too much time in our discussion on this topic. Anyone who has experience with an addictive substance or knows someone with a substance abuse problem knows how devastating these substances can be to overall health. The direct effect of the substance itself, combined with the alteration in good decision-making, rarely produces a healthy outcome in anyone under its influence. If you have ever seen the "before and after" pictures of individuals on certain addictive drugs like methamphetamines, you will immediately recognize how quickly their health deteriorates, along with what appears to be a rapid aging process.

Obviously, addictive drugs include prescription medications as well as some over-the-counter medications and foods. Any substance you feel you cannot do without and that would elicit an emotional and/or physical withdrawal if removed is a potential problem for you. This includes oxycodone, codeine, nicotine, steroids, diazepam (valium), sleeping medications, cough and cold medicines containing dextromethorphan, ADHD drugs, caffeine, alcohol, and a long list of illicit drugs including cocaine, heroin, methamphetamines, PCP, marijuana

(THC), LSD, and more. Some of these substances are more powerful than others; some are more addictive than others. The point is simply this: while there are extremely limited potential benefits from some of these substances in a highly managed clinical setting, as a lifestyle decision, addiction to any substance will result in poor, even fatal, outcomes. The fact that substance abuse and addiction are nearly always linked with other unhealthy and risky behaviors reinforces this notion.

The study of how various drug-like substances change genetic and protein expression is generally called pharmacogenomics. This is mostly involved in how new substances being tested for potential therapeutic benefit (as potential rescue interventions in our Lifestyle Synergy Model) might influence health outcomes. The same, however, is true of almost all of the addictive substances we listed above. Along with their well-known pharmaceutical effects (binding to receptors, inhibition of enzymes, etc.) and their toxic effects, many of these substances have been discovered to have genomic and epigenetic influences as well.[24,26,27] If you know you have (or think you have) a substance abuse or addiction, seek professional help to start the road to recovery right away. If you are making decisions under the influence of an addictive and controlling substance, you are rarely making good decisions.

Principle #6: Sexual promiscuity is fraught with physical and emotional consequences—a lifestyle of monogamy is the only healthy choice.

Common sense and biology tell us that a sexually transmitted disease (STD) cannot be passed between two disease-free, monogamous partners.[†] Unfortunately, STD research is so riddled with agendas, primarily driven by the fears of politicizing and moralizing a medical issue, that the basic facts are frequently obfuscated. Likewise, the opinion that monogamy is impractical or unlikely to be practiced should not dissuade us from making this basic recommendation. Whatever your views about politics or sexual behavior might be, the STD epidemic in the U.S. is simply overwhelming and can be considered a quintessential lifestyle-driven phenomenon.

---

† I realize there may be some exceptions to this rule involving other risky behaviors like sharing needles with individuals carrying the disease, having contact with an open sore, or, rarely, receiving blood transfusions.

According to the CDC, there were an estimated 19 million *new* STD infections in the U.S. in 2010 (ten times the 1.9 million new diabetes diagnoses that year), costing our healthcare system about $17 billion that year alone.[28] The lifetime implications of these diseases start very early as young people, who only represent 25% of the sexually experienced population in the United States, account for nearly half of all newly reported STDs. All totaled, it is estimated that over 65 million Americans currently live with some STD (would this qualify as a pandemic?).

As far back as 1990, a survey of female university students (seniors at the University of Michigan) showed that those women with five or more sexual partners were eight times more likely to report having an STD than those with only one partner, even after adjusting for age at first intercourse.[29] This relationship between the number of sexual partners and increased risk has held up in numerous populations and disease measurements.[30-33] The relationship between multiple sexual partners and the frequency of other risky behaviors is also a factor related to STD and other disease outcomes.[34]

In addition to the diseases themselves, which can be devastating and sometimes lethal, the burden of reduced fertility and long-term use of pharmaceutical drugs to limit STDs is difficult to measure. For instance, one of the most common STDs, gonorrhea, is caused by a bacterial infection that at one time was relatively easy to manage with antibiotics. Today, many strains of the bacterium *Neisseria gonorrhoeae* have become resistant to a host of our antibiotic medications such as sulfonilamides, penicillin, tetracycline, and ciprofloxacin. Researchers are becoming very concerned about the potential long-term consequences of continued drug resistance amongst once-treatable STD-causing organisms.[35] The additional burden upon our detoxification capacity and the destruction of our commensal (good) bacteria as we use higher doses and more powerful antibiotics are just more considerations in the battle against this growing lifestyle epidemic.

Here we agree with the CDC's advice: "*The most reliable ways to avoid infection with an STD are to abstain from sex (i.e., oral, vaginal, or anal sex) or to be in a long-term, mutually monogamous relationship with an uninfected partner.*"[36]

CHAPTER 14

A Purpose for Life—and a Community to Dwell

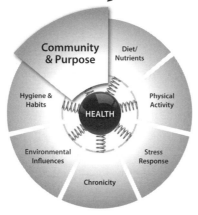

"A healthy body is the guest-chamber of the soul;
a sick body, its prison."

—Francis Bacon (1561–1626)

THROUGHOUT THIS BOOK WE have been describing what is, for many, a radically new way to view health and healthcare. Attempting to abandon the common diagnostic approach that emphasizes the disease rather than the patient, we have been advocating an approach that empowers individuals to change the lifestyle signals that coalesce into a synergistic health outcome. In this type of healthcare, the person, rather than their diagnosis, becomes the important and primary focus, including their history, their lifestyle decisions, their response to various therapies, and so on. But even as great a paradigm shift as this can be, it still doesn't fully encompass the whole human health condition. We are, after all, more than just physical beings but spiritual beings; more than individuals, we are a part of a larger community. Our overall health is dependent not only upon our personal lifestyle decisions, but also on how we understand our relationship with those around us—even about how we view our own purpose for living in the first place. In the final sphere of the Lifestyle Synergy Model, we want to explore how our understanding of who we are, our purpose for life, and the community with which we surround ourselves influences our well-being.

Principle #1: You exist for a purpose—you are no accident. Maintain your health in order to reach the fullness of your intended purpose.

If you are a parent, grandparent, aunt, or uncle you have probably had the opportunity to examine the artistic creativity of a young child. Sometimes they work for hours on a picture or even longer on a hunk of clay and plop it down into your lap and say, "Do you like it?" Of course, this is always easier to answer than the dreaded question, "Guess what it is?" Afraid to hurt their feelings, you ask a few innocent questions until they blurt out the answer, then you nod and tell them that it is one of the best pieces you have ever seen. A few years back, one of my children was learning the art of origami, an ancient Asian craft of folding a flat piece of paper into a three-dimensional object. As I was walking by, I noticed an exquisitely folded hat made from a large piece of paper and decided to model it for the household. At first it didn't fit perfectly but with a little pressure it conformed fairly well to my head. When I decided to show my daughter how good her hat looked on my head, her face quickly turned sour. As it turns out, ***the boat*** she was making wasn't quite finished, and now I had likely ruined it. A boat? I guess if you turned it the other way, it looked like a boat; but it wasn't obvious to me. You see, the beauty of an object might be in the eye of the beholder, but purpose and design are defined by its creator.

The prevailing scientific model tells us that human existence is at best a coincidence, at worst an accident. In fact, "purpose," as we might define it, has little place in the discussion of human existence, except perhaps as a means to transmit genetic material to the next generation.

Once your benefit to the fitness of the species is finished, we are told, your limited individual purpose fades away. Some scientists are quick to remind us that what appears to be "purpose" is merely an illusion. One of the great apologists for this position, Richard Dawkins, has said it this way: "*All appearances to the contrary, the only watchmaker in nature is the blind force of physics, albeit deployed in a very special way. A true watchmaker has foresight: he designs his cogs and springs, and plans their interconnections, with a future purpose in his mind's eye. Natural selection, the blind, unconscious automatic process which Darwin discovered, and which we now know is the explanation for the existence and apparently purposeful form of all life, has no purpose in mind. It has no mind and no mind's eye. It does not plan for the future. It has no vision, no foresight, no sight at all. If it can be said to play the role of watchmaker in nature, it is the blind watchmaker.*" He surmises: "*Biology is the study of complicated things that give the appearance of having been designed for a purpose.*"[1] In my opinion, this notion is comparable to men walking about with origami boats on their heads, insisting that we believe that their "hats" folded themselves from flat sheets of paper by coincidence.[†]

For me and many others, human purpose is defined by God, in whose image we are created. It is an intrinsic reality indelibly fixed to our very existence. It defines our relationship to God (as the pot owes its definition and purpose to the potter), but also defines our relationship to others, whose value and purpose are equally defined by the image of their Creator. It is, I am convinced, part of our conscience, something we can't fully remove even though we might try. Ironically, the younger generations of today, who have been taught that their biological existence is purposeless and accidental, are seeking meaning in life. They are "cause" driven because they have been starved of purpose.

When researchers attempt to define "purpose" and relate it to health outcomes, they have discovered a clear relationship. The definition they often use to describe purpose in life is the tendency to derive meaning from life's experiences and acquire a sense of intentionality and goal-directedness that guides behavior.[2] According to this definition, purpose

---

[†] I think the Apostle Paul, who found himself debating these same ideas in the shadow of the Parthenon in Athens (Acts 17:24–31), had this in mind when he wrote Romans 1:18–25.

in life is related to aspects of psychological health, including happiness, satisfaction, personal growth, and even better sleep. Results of a meta-analysis showed that a higher level of purpose in life was associated with better health, everyday competence, social integration, participation in the labor force, and socioeconomic status among middle-aged and older persons, and better treatment outcomes for persons with addiction. While there are limitations to creating prospective outcome trials based on purpose (as this can change over time), a focus of research has been elderly patients with dementia. In recent years, studies have shown that purpose in life and related aspects of well-being are associated with a substantially reduced risk of adverse cognitive health outcomes, including Alzheimer's disease (AD) and mild cognitive impairment, as well as a slower rate of cognitive decline even among older persons without AD or mild cognitive impairment. Purpose is also associated with a reduced risk of incident disability and death. Initial evidence suggests that purpose in life may also be modifiable, rendering it a potential treatment target.[2] In one particular study, 246 patients with AD were assessed via structured interviews and then examined postmortem. Those participants who reported higher levels of purpose in life exhibited higher cognitive function despite the burden of the disease. Furthermore, in examining whether purpose in life modified the association between pathologic effects of AD and the rate of cognitive decline, researchers found that higher levels of purpose in life reduced the effect of AD's pathologic changes upon cognitive decline.[2]

Purpose Defines Hope

Perhaps you have seen the posters or billboards of two women side-by-side. The one on the left is a young woman, perhaps in her early 20s, full of life, smiling. Next to her is another woman, disheveled, wrinkled, hollow-eyed, who looks to be about 50 years old. The billboard tells us that these are not two different women but the same woman only two years apart—before and after she becomes addicted to methamphetamines or crack cocaine. Look at the images in your mind—which one of these women thinks she has a future, which one sees purpose in her life, which one has hope? There are few things more devastating to the human condition than hopelessness. Without hope, investing any effort into tomorrow appears to have no value at all.

Those with no hope for the future are not sitting down to read the nutritional fact boxes to count the calories or determine whether there are trans-fats in their cookies. In fact, nearly all the recommendations in this book so far are of little consequence to those without hope and those with no sense of purpose. My prayer is that in the intricate discussion of how your decisions turn into health you will have seen the purposeful design that so many others missed and will choose to seek and maintain the purposeful relationship with God designed for you. In this way, your health will not become an end to itself but a means to pursue that great purpose for which you were created.

Principle # 2: Every day is a new day; if you have made poor decisions in the past, forgive yourself and move on to a better tomorrow.

As a corollary to our first principle, I want to encourage you not to give up. If you are like me, you have made a few mistakes in your life, and not a few unhealthy choices in the past. For many of you, the changes you need to make are difficult, and you may have failed on more than one occasion in the past. Don't give up hope. Forgive yourself and don't dwell on the failures of the past—tomorrow does not have to look like yesterday. Today is a new day.

Earlier we discussed how forgiveness of others can help us reduce anxiety and stress. When we hold a psychological debt from another person, it creates a root of bitterness that eats away at our own mental and physical health. Releasing this debt releases us from this burden. Believe it or not, forgiving others will add years to your life.[3] Likewise, if you hold yourself hostage to your own previous failures, you create a cycle of defeat and bitterness that is difficult to escape. Have you ever heard yourself say, "I know I should get healthier/start exercising/eat better, but I have tried it before and it didn't work"? Don't let your past dictate your future; you can move on—you have a purpose to pursue.

Perhaps you attempted to make all of your changes in just one sphere—only dietary changes or only exercise, for example. Now you realize that less radical changes in multiple spheres might be more effective and might even be easier to accomplish. Recall those things that have worked for you in the past, remove the reminders of your past failures, and set purposeful, hopeful, and realistic goals for your future health. Most likely you won't be able to do it alone; you will need a healthy community to help you make the changes.

Principle #3: Humans are intended to be in community. Invest yourself in others and let others invest in you—it will bring joy to the length of your days.

Humans are very complex social creatures. We can be defined by our family, tribe, language, culture, nationality, religion, race, or trade. We are born into some of these identity groups, while others we choose to join. Whether we like it or not, our lives and well-being are intertwined in some fashion by the groups we interact with or choose not to interact with. Scientists measure this in a generic way as a "sense of belonging." Those with a greater sense of belonging have a higher sense of self-worth, lower anxiety, and greater purpose, which translates into a greater sense of well-being and a higher likelihood of choosing healthier patterns of living. The opposite is true of those who intentionally shun social interactions. For over a decade we have known that those who choose to attend religious services regularly have a longer life expectancy than those who rarely or never do.[4] According to data published in 1999, this translates into a seven-year difference in life expectancy at age 20 between those who never attend and those who attend more than once a week. Further analysis appears to show greater benefit when religious activities are public rather than private and when those religions or denominations have specific codes of behavior that translate into healthy outcomes.[5] This doesn't mean that private spirituality is of little benefit; it just means that the social activities provided by interacting with others are a powerful part of how religious activities benefit our health.

Basic family dynamics also play a role in our health. As has been known for many years, marriage appears to increase life expectancy, especially in men.[6] Perhaps men make better health decisions when they sense increased purpose in their lives, or perhaps wives are helpful in curbing unhealthy behaviors in men.[†] Family stability also helps adolescents avoid poor lifestyle decisions. Parental divorce increases the likelihood of an adolescent choosing harmful behavior such as alcohol abuse, drug abuse, and promiscuity.[7-9] These behaviors are especially connected with negative feelings toward fathers through the divorce process.[10] Obviously you cannot change what your parents did or even what you have done in the past; but this information is an honest part of all the things you need to consider when attempting to leave the poor health patterns of the past and forge a new future. Many clinicians and patients are frustrated in their attempts to understand the driving force behind certain negative behavioral patterns; they would do well to ask questions about family dynamics, stress during childhood, and a "sense of belonging."

Principle #4: Lifestyle medicine is often best achieved with others. Find others with similar goals, and you will have better success.

Again, this principle is aligned very closely with the previous principle. If humans are intended to function within a strong social community, it is not surprising that health support groups and group therapy are proving to be strong tools of success for lifestyle-related therapies. Thankfully, this is also a great strategy to solve one of the biggest problems we currently face in our healthcare system: the lack of quality time available between clinicians and their patients. Group therapy can be as simple as getting a walking partner to make sure you keep up with your commitment to walk five times per week, or it can be an elaborate clinical program with a few dozen people. Regardless of how you define it, lifestyle changes are easier when they are reinforced by a social structure.

One of the positive new trends in healthcare is the use of group therapy for a broad range of interventions, but especially for weight management, diabetes prevention, depression, and cardiovascular risk reduction. It has been discovered that those involved with structured group therapy are less likely to drop out of the intervention and are

---

† I should note that cohabitation, which in many Western countries is increasingly replacing marriage, curiously does not change life expectancy in a manner different than being unmarried.

Are Online Social Networks Effective?

Today, social networking has a whole new definition. We can interact with hundreds or even thousands of "friends" online without ever meeting them face-to-face. Some, like myself, question the overall effect of this type of socialization on human health. Is it possible that internet socialization will have a less positive (or even a negative) health consequence? Not surprisingly, there is some research attempting to decipher the difference between traditional socialization and cyber-socialization. What appears to be emerging is that it depends on whether the Internet is being used to maintain a relationship that had been established in a traditional manner or whether the relationship itself was established and maintained through the Internet alone. Research tends to suggest that the latter form of cyber-socialization is less beneficial. This is especially true if Internet socialization time reduces a person's time spent communicating with family members or others in their traditional social network.[11-13]

Let's be clear, cyber-socializing is not going away—nor should it. There are numerous benefits from the information gained through the internet, especially in the area of health and lifestyle modification. If I wanted to find fifty different recipes to help me stay on a Mediterranean diet, they are just a few clicks away, along with videos to show me how to cook them. I can find groups of individuals with my specific condition I can chat with online to discuss my struggles and success stories.

What I am concerned about is that future generations may slowly abandon the traditional social formats, using cyber-social structures as their primary social interactions. If it turns out, as I would predict, that certain signals are obtained by social proximity (person-to-person or group dynamics), interactions performed exclusively online will diminish or eliminate them. We will certainly adapt to these changes, but we might have to wait a few years to find out what the cost of this adaptation might be.

much more likely to reach their goals.[14-16] In fact, the best weight-loss success appears to be through a combination of individual goal setting with some one-on-one sessions, combined with frequent and regular group sessions. These group sessions might focus on basic lifestyle interventions such as food selection (teaching about glycemic index for instance), cooking methods, exercise suggestions, and problem solving.

If you have had trouble reaching some of your lifestyle goals in the past, seek out a clinician who is capable of working to help you develop specific and reasonable goals—then pursue these goals within a group setting (even better if the same clinician provides that group setting). If you are unable to find any group that works for you, perhaps you can create one; or just find a willing companion who can come alongside you through the process. If that doesn't work, there are online groups with which you can share your progress. Many people find it rewarding to "post" their results (weight loss, test scores, exercise goals) in an online community set up to encourage healthy lifestyles. Lifestyle medicine, like life itself, is not meant to be accomplished alone.

Principle # 5: Celebrate with food, family, and friends. Don't abstain from all celebration because you are "on a diet"— celebrate responsibly and rejoice with those who rejoice.

This is the final principle of the chapter and also the final principle of the whole book—and it is a very important one. Sometimes when we are attempting to change our lives to become healthier we become very boring and negative people, perhaps only viewing our changes based on what we can't have (gluten-free, fat-free, low-carb, sugar-free, etc.). We restrict every aspect of our lives, and we sneer at those around us who don't hold themselves to our new "standard" of health.

This is no way to live. I want to encourage you to celebrate life. Yes, this means reasonable celebrations with family and friends for holidays, birthdays, and other special social occasions. These occasions not only allow for healthy social interactions, but if these are seasonal holiday events, they can also help calibrate our annual cycle of life. This isn't a license to overindulge for a month between Thanksgiving and New Year's Day, but it is a reflection on the fact that a healthy life should be regularly interrupted with celebration. In the biblical record, the people of God were told to gather three times in the year (coincident with agricultural gatherings) and commanded to rejoice; yes, commanded.[†] This rejoicing was always connected with a deep appreciation and gratefulness for the blessings they had received. Rejoicing and thankfulness should always be related; when we "rejoice" in the absence of thankfulness, our celebrations become self-indulgent and even harmful (reveling rather than rejoicing). One of the greatest lifestyle attributes you can possess is gratitude. When we really understand the blessings that are around us all the time, we can rejoice freely with others when they rejoice; we can celebrate without over-indulging; we can encourage those around us to be better; we can rejoice and be glad.

---

† The command to celebrate and rejoice is found in many passages connected to the three feast occasions, most notably in Deuteronomy 16 and Leviticus 23; the Psalms are a testament to the role of rejoicing and thanksgiving as regular parts of a healthy reflection upon the goodness provided to us by God.

CHAPTER 15

Epilogue: Can We Obtain Optimal Health?

"The practice of medicine is an art, not a trade;
a calling, not a business;
a calling in which your heart will be exercised
equally with your head. Often the best part
of your work will have nothing to do with
potions and powders, but with the exercise of
an influence of the strong upon the weak, of the righteous
upon the wicked, of the wise upon the foolish."
—Sir William Osler (1849-1919)

OUR HEALTH IS A priceless treasure, and many thieves conspire to plunder its wealth. How ironic that the safest storehouse designed to protect this treasure has its door wide open most of the time. We are definitely at a crossroads. The trillions of dollars we spend in healthcare and medical research each year are focused on the thief, not the open door. If only we had more money, scientists tell us, we could build better ways to protect ourselves against the disease intruder. What they don't realize is that a bigger and more sophisticated vault is no better than a flimsy tent if its door is left wide open. There must be a better way.

Throughout this book we have described what we think is the better way—the only real way to maintain our health and prevent the processes that lead to chronic disease. This doesn't mean, as some cynics might retort, that we should abandon all the medical technologies of the past few centuries and stop all future research. We aren't naïve enough to think that humans lived in some health utopia 200 years ago and that medical technology has taken all of that away. On the contrary, the past few centuries have witnessed many great advances that have allowed humankind to alleviate suffering in ways never previously conceived. We don't seek to go backward to a "good old day" that never was.

Instead, we suggest that the medical and technological advances of the past few centuries have permitted humans, especially in the West, to alter their lifestyle behaviors in a multitude of unhealthy ways. As we have catalogued throughout this book, most of these lifestyle changes have increased the chronic disease mechanisms in the body by stretching its physiological resilience and depleting its metabolic reserve, even leaving our genetic code with unhealthy tags so that each succeeding generation is progressively less healthy. According to this view, the medical advances of the recent past have actually enabled these unhealthy lifestyle changes to be perceived as having no consequence. Indeed, since many of these changes occurred gradually, the unintended consequences upon our health emerged gradually as well. When these changes have been adopted all at once, as in many developing nations, the consequences are more immediate and more devastating.

It is time to take lifestyle medicine seriously. The data is strong, the mechanisms are clear, and the stakes are too high to ignore. While we haven't yet arrived at Thomas Edison's prediction that "*The doctor of the future will give no medicine, but will interest her or his patients in the care of the human frame, in a proper diet, and in the cause and prevention of disease,*" I think we are a few steps closer. Even so, you don't have to wait until everyone else "gets it"; you can make a difference right now. But knowing what to do is not the same as doing it. If you are like me, more than half the battle is following through on what you already know to be true. Whether you are attempting to improve your own health or you are a healthcare provider facilitating the healing of others, the time to act is now.

Your DNA Is Not Your Destiny

Sequencing the human genome was an enormous accomplishment, one that promised to be the beginning of the end for all major diseases. If we could just connect each disease condition with its corresponding gene sequence, we would have the information necessary to reverse those diseases. Or so we thought.

There is no question that the techniques of molecular biology have been indispensable to our current understanding of human disease. As we have reviewed throughout this book, the information gained from genetics, genomics, and epigenetics has been crucial for our understanding of the powerful mechanisms hidden in the signals of our lifestyle decisions. Perhaps one of the greatest unexpected revelations gained from these studies is that our gene sequence is easily trumped by our gene expression. Your DNA is not your destiny. It may determine your health potential, but it cannot dictate your health outcome.

The signals you provide to your cells with each and every decision you make determine at least 80% of your health outcome. From the moment you awake to the time you choose to go to bed—each decision has a small impact. Will you eat breakfast, and if so, what will it be? How many hours will you spend sitting today? Will you give your spouse or your co-worker the benefit of the doubt or hold onto a grudge? When is your next thirty-minute walk or scheduled exercise? Can you get outside and get some sunlight, or will you spend the whole day in an artificial environment? Will you choose to pursue a greater purpose today or chalk it up as just another day? The choices are yours to make.

You are not a victim of genetics or circumstance. Your health is not dependent on those who control the government or the actuary controlling your insurance reimbursement. Your future is not dictated by your diagnosis; it is determined by your decisions. You will encounter obstacles in the road leading to your health goals. Will you view them as blessings to strengthen your perseverance and resolve or as curses that will derail you? Will you choose to invite others to help you navigate through them or go it alone and hope to survive? Your life is meaningful to someone else—do your decisions reflect that reality?

Can We Achieve Optimal Health?

When I contemplate the answer to this final question, I first ponder how one should define "optimal health." Do we mean by this that someone can live a disease-free existence if they play all their cards right? If so, then my answer would be "No." If, on the other hand, we mean that someone can live in such a way that their health rarely interferes with their purpose in life, then I would say "Yes"—you can achieve optimal health. It may be elusive, but it's not impossible.

The first part of finding optimal health is realizing that you have a purpose for living, and maintaining your health is one of the greatest ways to achieve that purpose, even when faced with great medical challenges. Two of the greatest mentors in my life faced tremendous health-related challenges; one suffered with rheumatoid arthritis from youth, and the other had his bladder removed in mid-life as a consequence of cancer. Both of them had a tremendous sense of calling and purpose, and both were fervent about their health. They understood that each decision they made (diet, physical activity, nutritional supplements, etc.) was allowing them to continue in the great purpose for which they were called. They each had a valid excuse to step aside and let other younger and healthier people take their place, but they stayed in the race until the end. Tens of thousands of people all over the world have been blessed by the teaching, preaching, and love they were able to impart *after* their illness had already taken its toll on their health. Optimal health, at times, was having just enough strength to sit on a chair and teach a room full of hungry disciples. I was just one of thousands honored to have received such a blessing.

It is in this spirit that I can say, unequivocally, that you can achieve optimal health. It doesn't mean that all your healthcare concerns will disappear, although many can and will when you implement a Lifestyle Synergy approach. What it does mean is that you can realize that your health is not an end, but a means to an end. There are, in fact, things more important than our own health, and we witness heroes willing to prove this each and every day. Most of us remember the heroic event of September 11th, when thousands of firefighters and police officers risked their health and their very lives for the sake of others. Volunteers entered the Fukushima nuclear power plant after the devastating tsunami of 2011, and optimizing their personal health was not the reason. These men and women were given international attention, but this kind of bravery and heroism happens every day in every nation. From anonymous kidney donors, to soldiers on the front lines, to mothers choosing to give up their remaining food in hopes that their starving children will survive until the next relief supply can arrive—health is a treasure we are willing to spend for the love of our children and the love of our neighbor. Thankfully, most of us don't have to make such choices. What, then, will you do with the blessing of good health?

Regardless of your situation, you have an opportunity to make a difference. My sincere hope is that you will always remain healthy enough to make a difference in the lives of others, and that you will be able to realize the full potential of your created purpose: body, soul, and spirit.

"I call heaven and earth to witness against you today, that I have set before you, life and death, the blessing and the curse. So choose life in order that you may live, you and your descendants, by loving the Lord your God, by obeying His voice, and by holding fast to Him; for this is your life and the length of your days..." Deuteronomy 30:19–20

REFERENCES

Chapter 2

1. CDC. Successes and opportunities for population-based prevention and control at a Glance 2011. 2011; http://www.cdc.gov/chronicdisease/resources/publications/AAG/ddt.htm.

2. CDC. Overweight and obesity - Health consequences. 2011; http://www.cdc.gov/obesity/causes/health.html.

3. Serdula M.K. et al. Prevalence of attempting weight loss and strategies for controlling weight. *JAMA*. 1999;282:1353-1358

4. WEIGHT-LOSS ADVERTISING: An analysis of current trends [Staff report]. 2002; http://www.ftc.gov/bcp/reports/weightloss.pdf.

5. Trus TL, Pope GD, Finlayson SR. National trends in utilization and outcomes of bariatric surgery. *Surgical Endoscopy*. May 2005;19(5):616-620.

6. Nguyen NT, Masoomi H, Magno CP, Nguyen XM, Laugenour K, Lane J. Trends in use of bariatric surgery, 2003-2008. *Journal of the American College of Surgeons*. Aug 2011; 213(2):261-266.

7. Haslam D, Rigby N. A long look at obesity. *Lancet*. Jul 10, 2010; 376(9735):85-86.

8. Haslam D. Obesity: A medical history. *Obes Rev*. 2007;8 Suppl 1:31-36.

9. Hensrud DD, Klein S. Extreme obesity. *Mayo Clin Proc*. 2006;81(10):5S-10S.

10. US Department of Health and Human Services, 1977.

11. US Department of Health and Human Services, 1996.

12. CDC. Overweight and obesity—Health consequences. 2011; http://www.cdc.gov/nchs/data/hestat/overweight/overweight_adult.htm.

13. Centre THaSCI. Statistics on obesity, physical activity and diet: England, 2010. 2010; http://www.ic.nhs.uk/webfiles/publications/opad10/Statistics_on_Obesity_Physical_Activity_and_Diet_England_2010.pdf.

14. MODI. Obesity in Australia. 2011; http://www.modi.monash.edu.au/obesity-facts-figures/obesity-in-australia/.

15. BBC. Obesity: In statistics. 2008; http://news.bbc.co.uk/2/hi/health/7151813.stm.

16. Yach D, Stuckler D, Brownell KD. Epidemiologic and economic consequences of the global epidemics of obesity and diabetes. *Nat Med*. 12:62-66.

17. Poston WS, II, Foreyt JP. Obesity is an environmental issue. *Atherosclerosis.* 1999;146:201-209.

18. Prentice AM. The emerging epidemic of obesity in developing countries. *International Journal of Epidemiology.* 2005;35(1):93-99.

19. Hossain P, Kawar B, El Nahas M. Obesity and diabetes in the developing world—a growing challenge. *N Engl J Med.* 2007;356:213-215.

20. Schulz LO. Effects of traditional and Western environments on prevalence of type 2 diabetes in Pima Indians in Mexico and the U.S. *Diabetes Care.* 2006;29(8):1866-1871.

21. Price RA, Charles MA, Pettitt DJ, Knowler WC. Obesity in Pima Indians: Large increases among post-World War II birth cohorts. *American Journal of Physical Anthropology.* Dec 1993;92(4):473-479.

22. Mokdad AH, Bowman BA, Ford ES, Vinicor F, Marks JS, Koplan JP. The continuing epidemics of obesity and diabetes in the United States. *JAMA.* 2001;286:1195-1200.

23. Wang Y, Beydoun MA, Liang L, Caballero B, Kumanyika SK. Will all Americans become overweight or obese? Estimating the progression and cost of the US obesity epidemic. *Obesity (Silver Spring).* 2008;16:2323-2330.

Chapter 3

1. Poston WSC, II, Foreyt JP. Obesity is an environmental issue. *Atherosclerosis.* 1999;146(2):201-209.

2. Wadden TA, Brownell KD, Foster GD. Obesity: Responding to the global epidemic. *Journal of Consulting and Clinical Psychology.* 2002;70(3):510-525.

3. Cordain L, Eaton SB, Sebastian A, et al. Origins and evolution of the Western diet: health implications for the 21st century. *Am J Clin Nutr.* 2005;81:341-354.

4. Levenstein H. *Revolution at the Table.* Berkeley: University of California Press; 2003.

5. Wilder L. I. *Farmer Boy.* New York: Harper Collins; 1933.

6. Krasner Khait B. The impact of refrigeration. http://www.history-magazine.com/refrig.html.

7. Wu JH, Miao W, Hu LG, Batist G. Identification and characterization of novel Nrf2 inducers designed to target the intervening region of Keap1. *Chem.Biol Drug Des.* 2010;75(5):475-480.

8. Cutler D, Glaeser EL, Shapiro JM. Why have Americans become more obese? *J of Economic Perspectives.* 2003;17(3):93-118.

9. Grotto D, Zied E. The standard American diet and its relationship to the health status of Americans. *Nutrition in Clinical Practice.* 2010;25(6):603-612.

10. Bray GA, Champagne CM. Beyond energy balance: There is more to obesity than kilocalories. *J Am Diet Assoc.* 2005;105(5, Supplement 1):17-23.

11. Putnam J, Allshouse J, Kantor, LS. US per capita food supply trends. *Food Review.* 2002;25(3).

12. Michael F. Jacobson PD. *Liquid Candy: How soft drinks are harming Americans' health.* Washington D.C.: Center for Science in the Public Interest; 2005.

13. Nicklas T, Baranowski T, Cullen KW, Berenson G. Eating patterns, dietary quality and obesity. *J Am Coll Nutr.* 2001;20(6):599-608.

14. St-Onge M-P, Keller KL, Heymsfield SB. Changes in childhood food consumption patterns: A cause for concern in light of increasing body weights. *Am J Clin Nutr.* 2003;78(6):1068-1073.

15. Soft Drinks Undermining Americans' Health. 1998. 2011: http://www.cspinet.org/new/soda_10_21_98.htm.

16. Nettleton JA, Lutsey PL, Wang Y, Lima JA, Michos ED, Jacobs DR, Jr. Diet soda intake and risk of incident metabolic syndrome and type 2 diabetes in the Multi-Ethnic Study of Atherosclerosis (MESA). *Diabetes Care.* Apr 2009;32(4):688-694.

17. Gardener H, Rundek T, Markert M, Wright CB, Elkind MS, Sacco RL. Diet soft drink consumption is associated with an increased risk of vascular events in the Northern Manhattan study. *J Gen Intern Med.* 2012;27:27.

18. Drewnowski A, Popkin BM. The nutrition transition: New trends in the global diet. *Nutr Rev.* Feb 1997;55(2):31-43.

19. Simopoulos AP. Evolutionary aspects of diet, the omega-6/omega-3 ratio and genetic variation: Nutritional implications for chronic diseases. *Biomed Pharmacother.* 2006;60(9):502-507.

20. Gillman MW, Rifas-Shiman SL, Frazier AL, et al. Family dinner and diet quality among older children and adolescents. *Arch fam med.* Mar 2000;9(3):235-240.

21. Biing-Hwan Lin JG, and Frazão E. Nutrient contribution of food away from home. Washington DC: Economic Research Services, US Dept of Agriculture; 1999:231-242.

22. Lin B GJ, Frazao E. Popularity of dining out presents barrier to dietary improvements. *Food Rev.* 1998:2-10.

23. Forthun L. *Family nutrition: The truth about family meals*: University of Florida IFAS Extension;2008.

24. Gardyn R. Convenience. *American Demographics.* 2002;24(3):30-33.

25. Jabs J, Devine C. Time scarcity and food choices: An overview. *Appetite.* 2006;47(2):196-204.

26. Guthrie JF, Lin BH, Frazao E. Role of food prepared away from home in the American diet, 1977-78 versus 1994-96: Changes and consequences. *Journal of nutrition education and behavior.* 2002;34(3):140-150.

27. Popkin BM. Global nutrition dynamics: The world is shifting rapidly toward a diet linked with noncommunicable diseases. *Am J Clin Nutr.* 2006;84:289-298.

28. Hill H. Food miles - background and marketing. In: Service NSAI, ed2008.

29. Cowan RS. The "Industrial Revolution" in the home: Household technology and social change in the 20th century. *Technology and culture.* Jan 1976;17(1):1-23.

30. Lanningham-Foster L, Nysse LJ, Levine JA. Labor saved, calories lost: The energetic impact of domestic labor-saving devices. *Obes Res.* Oct 2003;11(10):1178-1181.

31. Salmon J ON, Bauman A, Schmitz MK, Booth M. Leisure-time, occupational, and household physical activity among professional, skilled, and less-skilled workers and homemakers. *Prev Med.* 2000;30(3):191-199.

32. Statistics BoL. American Time Use Survey—2008 results. In: Labor USDo, ed2008.

33. Pate RR PM, Blair SN, et al. Physical activity and public health. A recommendation from the CDC and the American College of Sports Medicine. *JAMA.* 1995;273(5):402-407.

34. CDC. U.S. physical activity statistics. In: Statistics. NCfH, ed2009.

35. Brownson R, Boehmer TK, Luke DA. Declining rates of physical activity in the U.S.: What are the contributors? *Annu Rev Public Health* 2005;26:421-443.

36. Egger, GJ, Vogels, N, Westerterp, KR. Estimating historical changes in physical activity levels. Med J Aust 2001;175: 635–636.

37. Lundin A LI, Hallsten L, Ottosson J, Hemmingsson T. Unemployment and mortality—a longitudinal prospective study on selection and causation in 49321 Swedish middle-aged men. *J Epidemiol Community Health.* 2010;64(1):22-28.

38. Van Domelen DR, Koster A, Caserotti P, et al. Employment and physical activity in the U.S. *American J Prev Med.* 2011;41(2):136-145.

39. Matthews CE, Chen KY, Freedson PS, et al. Amount of time spent in sedentary behaviors in the United States, 2003-2004. *Am J Epidemiol.* 2008;167(7):875-881.

40. fcc.gov. http://transition.fcc.gov/Bureaus/Mass_Media/Factsheets/factvchip.html.

41. Fine, Ben (1999) "Household Appliances and the Use of Time: The United States and Britain since the 1920s. A Comment." *Economic History Review*, 52 (3). pp. 552-562.

42. www.aacap.org/cs/root/facts_for_families/children_and_watching_tv.

43. Tucker LA, Tucker JM. Television viewing and obesity in 300 women: Evaluation of the pathways of energy intake and physical activity. *Obesity.* 2011;19(10). Epub.

44. Dietz WH, Jr., Gortmaker SL. Do we fatten our children at the television set? Obesity and television viewing in children and adolescents. *Pediatrics.* May 1985;75(5):807-812.

45. Dietz WH. The role of lifestyle in health: The epidemiology and consequences of inactivity. *Proc Nutr Soc.* 1996;55:829-840.

46. Gottlieb DJ, Punjabi NM, Newman AB, et al. Association of sleep time with diabetes mellitus and impaired glucose tolerance. *Arch Intern Med.* Apr 25, 2005;165(8):863-867.

47. Knutson KL, Van Cauter E, Rathouz PJ, DeLeire T, Lauderdale DS. Trends in the prevalence of short sleepers in the USA: 1975-2006. *Sleep.* 2010;33(1):37-45.

48. Kuriyan R, Bhat S, Thomas T, Vaz M, Kurpad AV. Television viewing and sleep are associated with overweight among urban and semi-urban South Indian children. *Nutrition Journal.* 2007;6:25.

49. Garaulet M, Ortega FB, Ruiz JR, et al. Short sleep duration is associated with increased obesity markers in European adolescents: Effect of physical activity and dietary habits. The HELENA study. *Int J Obes.* 2011; 35(10):1308-17.

50. Kripke DF, Langer RD, Kline LE. Hypnotics' association with mortality or cancer: A matched cohort study. *BMJ Open.* 2012;2(1) e000850.

Chapter 4

1. Simon RR, Marks V, Leeds AR, Anderson JW. A comprehensive review of oral glucosamine use and effects on glucose metabolism in normal and diabetic individuals. *Diabetes Metab Res Rev.* Jan 2011;27(1):14-27.

2. Elder CR, Gullion CM, Funk KL, Debar LL, Lindberg NM, Stevens VJ. Impact of sleep, screen time, depression and stress on weight change in the intensive weight loss phase of the LIFE study. *Int J Obes (Lond).* Jan 2012;36(1):86-92.

3. Jiang R, Manson JE, Stampfer MJ, Liu S, Willett WC, Hu FB. Nut and peanut butter consumption and risk of type 2 diabetes in women. *JAMA.* Nov 27, 2002;288(20):2554-2560.

4. Eslick GD, Howe PR, Smith C, Priest R, Bensoussan A. Benefits of fish oil supplementation in hyperlipidemia: A systematic review and meta-analysis. *Int J Cardiol.* Jul 24, 2009;136(1):4-16.

5. Clegg DO, Reda DJ, Harris CL, et al. Glucosamine, chondroitin sulfate, and the two in combination for painful knee osteoarthritis. *N Engl J Med.* 2006;354(8):795-808.

Chapter 5

1. McNutt WF. Vis Medicatrix Naturae. *Cal State J Med.* Dec 1923;21(12):510-511.

2. Reynolds RM, Dennison EM, Walker BR, et al. Cortisol secretion and rate of bone loss in a population-based cohort of elderly men and women. *Calcif Tissue Int.* Sep 2005;77(3):134-138.

3. Fries E, Dettenborn L, Kirschbaum C. The cortisol awakening response (CAR): Facts and future directions. *Int.J Psychophysiol.* 2009;72(1):67-73.

4. Thayer JF, Yamamoto SS, Brosschot JF. The relationship of autonomic imbalance, heart rate variability and cardiovascular disease risk factors. *Int J Cardiol.* May 28, 2010;141(2):122-131.

5. Thayer JF, Ahs F, Fredrikson M, Sollers JJ, 3rd, Wager TD. A meta-analysis of heart rate variability and neuroimaging studies: Implications for heart rate variability as a marker of stress and health. *Neurosci Biobehav Rev.* Feb 2012;36(2):747-756.

6. Stolarz K, Staessen JA, Kuznetsova T, et al. Host and environmental determinants of heart rate and heart rate variability in four European populations. *J Hypertens.* Mar 2003;21(3):525-535.

7. Kagan VE, Shvedova A, Serbinova E, et al. Dihydrolipoic acid—a universal antioxidant both in the membrane and in the aqueous phase. Reduction of peroxyl, ascorbyl and chromanoxyl radicals. *Biochem Pharmacol.* 1992;44(8):1637-1649.

8. DeFronzo RA, Abdul-Ghani MA. Preservation of beta-cell function: The key to diabetes prevention. *J Clin Endocrinol Metab.* Aug 2011;96(8):2354-2366.

9. Winsloe C, Earl S, Dennison EM, Cooper C, Harvey NC. Early life factors in the pathogenesis of osteoporosis. *Curr Osteoporos Rep.* Dec 2009;7(4):140-144.

10. Knowler WC, Barrett-Connor E, Fowler SE, et al. Reduction in the incidence of type 2 diabetes with lifestyle intervention or metformin. *N Engl J Med.* Feb 7, 2002;346(6):393-403.

11. Knowler WC, Fowler SE, Hamman RF, et al. 10-year follow-up of diabetes incidence and weight loss in the Diabetes Prevention Program Outcomes Study. *Lancet.* Nov 14, 2009;374(9702):1677-1686.

12. Hivert MF, Jablonski KA, Perreault L, et al. Updated genetic score based on 34 confirmed type 2 diabetes Loci is associated with diabetes incidence and regression to normoglycemia in the diabetes prevention program. *Diabetes.* Apr 2011;60(4):1340-1348.

Chapter 6

1. Friedman RC, Farh KK, Burge CB, Bartel DP. Most mammalian mRNAs are conserved targets of microRNAs. *Genome Res.* Jan 2009;19(1):92-105.

2. Wang Z. MicroRNA: A matter of life or death. *World J Biol Chem.* Apr 26 2010;1(4):41-54.

3. Jayawardena TM, Egemnazarov B, Finch EA, et al. MicroRNA-mediated in vitro and in vivo direct reprogramming of cardiac fibroblasts to cardiomyocytes. *Circ Res.* May 25, 2012;110(11):1465-1473.

4. Dolinoy DC. The agouti mouse model: An epigenetic biosensor for nutritional and environmental alterations on the fetal epigenome. *Nutr Rev.* Aug 2008;66 Suppl 1:7S-11S.

5. Ng SF, Lin RC, Laybutt DR, Barres R, Owens JA, Morris MJ. Chronic high-fat diet in fathers programs beta-cell dysfunction in female rat offspring. *Nature.* Oct 21, 2010;467(7318):963-966.

6. Wei J, Lin Y, Li Y, et al. Perinatal exposure to bisphenol A at reference dose predisposes offspring to metabolic syndrome in adult rats on a high-fat diet. *Endocrinology.* Aug 2011;152(8):3049-3061.

7. Lim U, Song MA. Dietary and lifestyle factors of DNA methylation. *Methods Mol Biol.* 2012;863:359-376.

8. Hyson DA. A comprehensive review of apples and apple components and their relationship to human health. *Adv Nutr.* Sep 2011;2(5):408-420.

9. Gerhauser C. Cancer chemopreventive potential of apples, apple juice, and apple components. *Planta Med.* Oct 2008;74(13):1608-1624.

10. Boyer J, Liu RH. Apple phytochemicals and their health benefits. *Nutrition Journal.* May 12, 2004;3:5.

11. Boots AW, Haenen GR, Bast A. Health effects of quercetin: From antioxidant to nutraceutical. *Eur J Pharmacol.* May 13, 2008;585(2-3):325-337.

12. *The Science of Flavonoids.* New York: Springer; 2006.

13. *Flavonoids in Health and Disease, Second Edition (Antioxidants in Health and Disease)* Second ed. New York: Marcel Dekker Inc.; 2003.

14. Jung CH, Cho I, Ahn J, Jeon TI, Ha TY. Quercetin reduces high-fat diet-induced fat accumulation in the liver by regulating lipid metabolism genes. *Phytother Res.* Mar 23, 2012.

15. Notas G, Nifli AP, Kampa M, et al. Quercetin accumulates in nuclear structures and triggers specific gene expression in epithelial cells. *J Nutr Biochem.* Jul 20, 2011; 23(6):656-66.

16. Gao X, Cassidy A, Schwarzschild MA, Rimm EB, Ascherio A. Habitual intake of dietary flavonoids and risk of Parkinson disease. *Neurology.* Apr 10, 2012;78(15):1138-1145.

17. McCullough ML, Peterson JJ, Patel R, Jacques PF, Shah R, Dwyer JT. Flavonoid intake and cardiovascular disease mortality in a prospective cohort of US adults. *Am J Clin Nutr.* Feb 2012;95(2):454-464.

18. Clere N, Faure S, Martinez MC, Andriantsitohaina R. Anticancer properties of flavonoids: Roles in various stages of carcinogenesis. *Cardiovasc Hematol Agents Med Chem.* Apr 1, 2011;9(2):62-77.

19. Prasain JK, Carlson SH, Wyss JM. Flavonoids and age-related disease: Risk, benefits and critical windows. *Maturitas.* Jun 2010;66(2):163-171.

20. Sawan C, Vaissiere T, Murr R, Herceg Z. Epigenetic drivers and genetic passengers on the road to cancer. *Mutat Res.* July 2008; 642(1-2): 1-13.

Chapter 7

1. Franz MJ, VanWormer JJ, Crain AL, et al. Weight-loss outcomes: A systematic review and meta-analysis of weight-loss clinical trials with a minimum 1-year follow-up. *J Am Diet Assoc.* Oct 2007;107(10):1755-1767.

2. Thomas RJ, Kottke TE, Brekke MJ, et al. Attempts at changing dietary and exercise habits to reduce risk of cardiovascular disease: Who's doing what in the community? *Prev Cardiol.* Summer 2002;5(3):102-108.

3. Chiuve SE, Fung TT, Rexrode KM, et al. Adherence to a low-risk, healthy lifestyle and risk of sudden cardiac death among women. *JAMA.* Jul 6, 2011;306(1):62-69.

4. Knowler WC, Barrett-Connor E, Fowler SE, et al. Reduction in the incidence of type 2 diabetes with lifestyle intervention or metformin. *N Engl J Med.* Feb 7, 2002;346(6):393-403.

5. Knowler WC, Fowler SE, Hamman RF, et al. 10-year follow-up of diabetes incidence and weight loss in the Diabetes Prevention Program Outcomes Study. *Lancet.* Nov 14, 2009;374(9702):1677-1686.

Chapter 8

1. Schulze MB HK, Manson JE, Willett WC, Meigs JB, Weikert C, Heidemann C, Colditz GA, and Hu FB. Dietary pattern, inflammation, and incidence of type 2 diabetes in women. *Am J Clin Nutr* 2005;82(3):675-684.

2. Van Dam RM, Rimm EB, Willett WC, Stampfer MJ, Hu FB. Dietary patterns and risk for type 2 diabetes mellitus in U.S. men. *Ann Intern Med.* Feb 5, 2002;136(3):201-209.

3. Keys A AC, Blackburn HW, et al. Epidemiological studies related to coronary heart disease: Characteristics of men aged 40-59 in seven countries. *Acta Med Scand Suppl.* 1966;460:1-392.

4. Keys A GF. Dietary fat and serum cholesterol. *Am J Public Health.* 1957;47:1520-1530.

5. Keys A, Menotti A, Karvonen MJ, et al. The diet and 15-year death rate in the seven countries study. *Am J Epidemiol.* Dec 1986;124(6):903-915.

6. Willett WC. *Eat, Drink and Be Healthy.* New York; Free Press; 2001.

7. Hu FB WW. Optimal diets for prevention of coronary heart disease. *JAMA.* 2002;288(20):2569-2578.

8. Hu FB MJ, Willett WC. Types of dietary fat and risk of coronary heart disease: A critical review. *J Am Coll Nutr.* 2001;20(1):5-19.

9. Chiuve SE, Fung TT, Rexrode KM, et al. Adherence to a low-risk, healthy lifestyle and risk of sudden cardiac death among women. *JAMA.* Jul 6 2011;306(1):62-69.

10. Sofi F, Cesari F, Abbate R, Gensini GF, Casini A. Adherence to Mediterranean diet and health status: Meta-analysis. *BMJ.* 2008;337:a1344.

11. Sofi F, Abbate R, Gensini GF, Casini A. Accruing evidence on benefits of adherence to the Mediterranean diet on health: An updated systematic review and meta-analysis. *Am J Clin Nutr.* Nov 2010;92(5):1189-1196.

12. Mena MP, Sacanella E, Vazquez-Agell M, et al. Inhibition of circulating immune cell activation: A molecular antiinflammatory effect of the Mediterranean diet. *Am J Clin Nutr.* 2008;89(1):248-256.

13. Andrade AM, Greene GW, Melanson KJ. Eating slowly led to decreases in energy intake within meals in healthy women. *J Am Diet Assoc.* Jul 2008;108(7):1186-1191.

14. Hsieh SD, Muto T, Murase T, Tsuji H, Arase Y. Eating until feeling full and rapid eating both increase metabolic risk factors in Japanese men and women. *Public health nutrition.* Feb 3, 2011:1-4.

15. Takayama S, Akamine Y, Okabe T, et al. Rate of eating and body weight in patients with type 2 diabetes or hyperlipidaemia. *Jrnl Int Med Res.* Jul-Aug 2002;30(4):442-444.

16. Grotto D, Zied E. The standard American diet and its relationship to the health status of Americans. *Nutrition in Clinical Practice.* 2010;25(6):603-612.

17. Young LR, Nestle M. The contribution of expanding portion sizes to the US obesity epidemic. *Am J Public Health.* Feb 2002;92(2):246-249.

18. Ello-Martin JA, Ledikwe JH, Rolls BJ. The influence of food portion size and energy density on energy intake: Implications for weight management. *Am J Clin Nutr.* Jul 2005;82(1 Suppl):236S-241S.

19. Vermeer WM, Steenhuis IH, Leeuwis FH, Heymans MW, Seidell JC. Small portion sizes in worksite cafeterias: Do they help consumers to reduce their food intake? *International Journal of Obesity (2005).* Sep 2011;35(9):1200-1207.

20. Spill MK, Birch LL, Roe LS, Rolls BJ. Eating vegetables first: The use of portion size to increase vegetable intake in preschool children. *Am J Clin Nutr.* May 2010;91(5):1237-1243.

21. Rolls BJ, Roe LS, Meengs JS. Portion size can be used strategically to increase vegetable consumption in adults. *Am J Clin Nutr.* Apr 2010;91(4):913-922.

22. Horikawa C, Kodama S, Yachi Y, et al. Skipping breakfast and prevalence of overweight and obesity in Asian and Pacific regions: A meta-analysis. *Prev Med.* Oct 2011;53(4-5):260-267.

23. Betts JA, Thompson D, Richardson JD, et al. Bath Breakfast Project (BBP)—examining the role of extended daily fasting in human energy balance and associated health outcomes: Study protocol for a randomised controlled trial [ISRCTN31521726]. *Trials.* 2011;12:172.

24. Pereira MA, Erickson E, McKee P, et al. Breakfast frequency and quality may affect glycemia and appetite in adults and children. *J Nutr.* Jan 2011;141(1):163-168.

25. Ludwig DS, Majzoub JA, Al-Zahrani A, Dallal GE, Blanco I, Roberts SB. High glycemic index foods, overeating, and obesity. *Pediatrics.* Mar 1999;103(3):E26.

26. Warren JM, Henry CJ, Simonite V. Low glycemic index breakfasts and reduced food intake in preadolescent children. *Pediatrics.* Nov 2003;112(5):E414.

27. Campbell SM. Hydration needs throughout the lifespan. *J Am Coll Nutr.* Oct 2007;26(5 Suppl):585S-587S.

28. Sawka MN, Cheuvront SN, Carter R, 3rd. Human water needs. *Nutr Rev.* Jun 2005;63(6 Pt 2):S30-39.

29. Bray GA, Nielsen SJ, Popkin BM. Consumption of high-fructose corn syrup in beverages may play a role in the epidemic of obesity. *Am J Clin Nutr.* Apr 2004;79(4):537-543.

30. Ludwig DS, Peterson KE, Gortmaker SL. Relation between consumption of sugar-sweetened drinks and childhood obesity: A prospective, observational analysis. *Lancet.* Feb 17, 2001;357(9255):505-508.

31. Malik VS, Schulze MB, Hu FB. Intake of sugar-sweetened beverages and weight gain: A systematic review. *Am J Clin Nutr.* Aug 2006;84(2):274-288.

32. Gibson S. Sugar-sweetened soft drinks and obesity: A systematic review of the evidence from observational studies and interventions. *Nutr Res Rev.* Dec 2008;21(2):134-147.

33. Libuda L, Kersting M. Soft drinks and body weight development in childhood: Is there a relationship? *Curr Opin Clin Nutr Metab Care.* Nov 2009;12(6):596-600.

34. USDA. http://ndb.nal.usda.gov/ndb/foods/list.

35. Valtin H. "Drink at least eight glasses of water a day." Really? Is there scientific evidence for "8 x 8"? *Am J Physiol Regul Integr Comp Physiol.* Nov 2002;283(5):R993-1004.

36. Kong A, Beresford SA, Alfano CM, et al. Associations between snacking and weight loss and nutrient intake among postmenopausal overweight to obese women in a dietary weight-loss intervention. *J Am Diet Assoc.* Dec 2011;111(12):1898-1903.

Chapter 9

1. Morrato EH, Hill JO, Wyatt HR, Ghushchyan V, Sullivan PW. Physical activity in U.S. adults with diabetes and at risk for developing diabetes, 2003. *Diabetes Care.* Feb 2007;30(2):203-209.

2. Sieverdes JC, Sui X, Lee DC, et al. Physical activity, cardiorespiratory fitness and the incidence of type 2 diabetes in a prospective study of men. *Br J Sports Med.* 2009;44(4):238-244.

3. Blair SN, LaMonte MJ, Nichaman MZ. The evolution of physical activity recommendations: How much is enough? *Am J Clin Nutr.* May 2004;79(5):913S-920S.

4. Van Domelen DR, Koster A, Caserotti P, et al. Employment and physical activity in the U.S. *Am J Prev Med.* 2011;41(2):136-145.

5. Matthews CE, Chen KY, Freedson PS, et al. Amount of time spent in sedentary behaviors in the United States, 2003-2004. *Am J Epidemiol.* 2008;167(7):875-881.

6. Dietz WH. The role of lifestyle in health: The epidemiology and consequences of inactivity. *Proc Nutr Soc.* 1996;55:829-840.

7. Tucker LA, Tucker JM. Television viewing and obesity in 300 women: Evaluation of the pathways of energy intake and physical activity. *Obesity.* 2011;19(10). Epub.

8. Morris JN, Heady JA, Raffle PAB, Roberts CG, Parks JW. Coronary heart disease and physical activity of work. *The Lancet.* 1953;262(6796):1111-1120.

9. Pinto Pereira SM, Ki M, Power C. Sedentary behaviour and biomarkers for cardiovascular disease and diabetes in mid-life: The role of television-viewing and sitting at work. *PloS One.* 2012;7(2):e31132.

10. Dunstan DW, Thorp AA, Healy GN. Prolonged sitting: Is it a distinct coronary heart disease risk factor? *Curr Opin Cardiol.* Sep 2011;26(5):412-419.

11. Van der Ploeg HP, Chey T, Korda RJ, Banks E, Bauman A. Sitting time and all-cause mortality risk in 222 497 Australian adults. *Arch Intern Med.* March 26, 2012;172(6):494-500.

12. Pate RR, Mitchell JA, Byun W, Dowda M. Sedentary behaviour in youth. *Br J Sports Med.* Sep 2011;45(11):906-913.

13. Proper KI, Singh AS, van Mechelen W, Chinapaw MJ. Sedentary behaviors and health outcomes among adults: A systematic review of prospective studies. *Am J Prev Med.* Feb 2011;40(2):174-182.

14. Shoham N, Gottlieb R, Sharabani-Yosef O, Zaretsky U, Benayahu D, Gefen A. Static mechanical stretching accelerates lipid production in 3T3-L1 adipocytes by activating the MEK signaling pathway. *American Journal of Physiology. Cell Physiology.* Jan 2012;302(2):C429-441.

15. Dunstan DW, Kingwell BA, Larsen R, et al. Breaking up prolonged sitting reduces postprandial glucose and insulin responses. *Diabetes Care.* Feb 28, 2012;35(5):976-83.

16. Wen CP, Wai JP, Tsai MK, et al. Minimum amount of physical activity for reduced mortality and extended life expectancy: A prospective cohort study. *Lancet.* Oct 1, 2011;378(9798):1244-1253.

17. Chiuve SE, Fung TT, Rexrode KM, et al. Adherence to a low-risk, healthy lifestyle and risk of sudden cardiac death among women. *JAMA.* Jul 6, 2011;306(1):62-69.

18. Boone-Heinonen J, Evenson KR, Taber DR, Gordon-Larsen P. Walking for prevention of cardiovascular disease in men and women: A systematic review of observational studies. *Obesity Reviews.* 2009;10(2):204-217.

19. Knowler WC, Barrett-Connor E, Fowler SE, et al. Reduction in the incidence of type 2 diabetes with lifestyle intervention or metformin. *N Engl J Med.* Feb 7, 2002;346(6):393-403.

20. Weinstock RS, Brooks G, Palmas W, et al. Lessened decline in physical activity and impairment of older adults with diabetes with telemedicine and pedometer use: Results from the IDEATel study. *Age and Ageing.* 2010;40(1):98-105.

21. Shenoy S, Guglani R, Sandhu JS. Effectiveness of an aerobic walking program using heart rate monitor and pedometer on the parameters of diabetes control in Asian Indians with type 2 diabetes. *Primary Care Diabetes.* 2010;4(1):41-45.

22. Walking: Trim your waistline, improve your health. http://www.mayoclinic.com/health/walking/HQ01612. Accessed May 7, 2012.

23. Nygaard H, Tomten SE, Høstmark AT. Slow postmeal walking reduces postprandial glycemia in middle-aged women. *Appl Physio Nutr Metab.* 2009;34(6):1087-1092.

24. Lakka TA, Laaksonen DE. Physical activity in prevention and treatment of the metabolic syndrome. *Appl Physio Nutr Metab* Feb 2007;32(1):76-88.

25. Borghouts LB, Keizer HA. Exercise and insulin sensitivity: A review. *Int J Sports Med.* Jan 2000;21(1):1-12.

26. Exercise and Type 2 Diabetes: American College of Sports Med.: Medicine & Science in Sports & Exercise. 2012.

27. Statement on Exercise: Benefits and Recommendations for Physical Activity Programs for All Americans: A Statement for Health Professionals by the Committee on Exercise and Cardiac Rehabilitation of the Council on Clinical Cardiology, American Heart Association. 2012.

28. Friedenreich CM, Neilson HK, Woolcott CG, et al. Inflammatory marker changes in a yearlong randomized exercise intervention trial among postmenopausal women. *Cancer Prev Res (Phila).* Jan 2012;5(1):98-108.

29. Marcus RL, Smith S, Morrell G, et al. Comparison of combined aerobic and high-force eccentric resistance exercise with aerobic exercise only for people with type 2 diabetes mellitus. *Phys Ther.* Nov 2008;88(11):1345-1354.

30. Moreira SR, Simoes GC, Moraes JF, Motta DF, Campbell CS, Simoes HG. Blood glucose control for individuals with type-2 diabetes: Acute effects of resistance exercise of lower cardiovascular-metabolic stress. *J Strength Cond Res.* Nov 29, 2011. Epub.

31. MacLean PS, Zheng D, Dohm GL. Muscle glucose transporter (GLUT 4) gene expression during exercise. *Exerc Sport Sci Rev.* Oct 2000;28(4):148-152.

32. Hood DA. Mechanisms of exercise-induced mitochondrial biogenesis in skeletal muscle. *Appl Physio Nutr Metab.* Jun 2009;34(3):465-472.

33. McGee SL, Hargreaves M. Histone modifications and exercise adaptations. *J Appl Physiol.* Jan 2011;110(1):258-263.

34. Hawley JA, Burke LM, Phillips SM, Spriet LL. Nutritional modulation of training-induced skeletal muscle adaptations. *J Appl Physiol.* Mar 2011;110(3):834-845.

35. Janssen I, Ross R. Vigorous intensity physical activity is related to the metabolic syndrome independent of the physical activity dose. *Int J Epidemiol.* Mar 24, 2012. Epub.

36. Perry CG, Heigenhauser GJ, Bonen A, Spriet LL. High-intensity aerobic interval training increases fat and carbohydrate metabolic capacities in human skeletal muscle. *Appl Physio Nutr Metab.* Dec 2008;33(6):1112-1123.

37. Yamaguchi W, Fujimoto E, Higuchi M, Tabata I. A DIGE proteomic analysis for high-intensity exercise-trained rat skeletal muscle. *J Biochem.* Sep 2010;148(3):327-333.

38. Fujimoto E, Machida S, Higuchi M, Tabata I. Effects of nonexhaustive bouts of high-intensity intermittent swimming training on GLUT-4 expression in rat skeletal muscle. *J Physiol Sci.* Mar 2010;60(2):95-101.

39. Juvancic-Heltzel JA, Glickman EL, Barkley JE. The effect of variety on physical activity: A cross-sectional study. *J Strength Cond Res.* Mar 5, 2012. Epub.

40. Harmel K. Adding variety to an exercise routine helps increase adherence. 2000; http://news.ufl.edu/2000/10/24/variety/. Accessed May 7, 2012.

41. Podewils LJ, Guallar E, Kuller LH, et al. Physical activity, APOE genotype, and dementia risk: Findings from the Cardiovascular Health Cognition Study. *Am J Epidemiol.* Apr 1, 2005;161(7):639-651.

42. Kawasaki T, Sullivan CV, Ozoe N, Higaki H, Kawasaki J. A long-term, comprehensive exercise program that incorporates a variety of physical activities improved the blood pressure, lipid and glucose metabolism, arterial stiffness, and balance of middle-aged and elderly Japanese. *Hypertens Res.* Sep 2011;34(9):1059-1066.

43. Thompson Coon J, Boddy K, Stein K, Whear R, Barton J, Depledge MH. Does participating in physical activity in outdoor natural environments have a greater effect on physical and mental wellbeing than physical activity indoors? A systematic review. *Environ Sci Technol.* Mar 1, 2011;45(5):1761-1772.

44. Balagué F, Mannion AF, Pellisé F, Cedraschi C. Non-specific low back pain. *The Lancet.* 2012;379:482-491.

45. Burdorf A, Naaktgeboren B, de Groot HC. Occupational risk factors for low back pain among sedentary workers. *J Occup Med.* Dec 1993;35(12):1213-1220.

46. Shiri R, Karppinen J, Leino-Arjas P, Solovieva S, Viikari-Juntura E. The association between obesity and low back pain: A meta-analysis. *Am J Epidemiol.* Jan 15, 2010;171(2):135-154.

47. Hoiriis KT, Pfleger B, McDuffie FC, et al. A randomized clinical trial comparing chiropractic adjustments to muscle relaxants for subacute low back pain. *J Manipulative Physiol Ther.* 2004;27(6):388-398.

48. Smart LJ, Jr., Smith DL. Postural dynamics: Clinical and empirical implications. *J Manipulative Physiol Ther.* Jun 2001;24(5):340-349.

49. Kritz MF, Cronin J. Static posture assessment screen of athletes: Benefits and considerations. *Strength and Conditioning Journal.* 2008;30(5):18-27.

50. Hrysomallis C, Goodman C. A review of resistance exercise and posture realignment. *J Strength Cond Res.* 2001;15(3):385-390.

51. Novak CB. Upper extremity work-related musculoskeletal disorders: A treatment perspective. *J Orthop Sports Phys Ther.* 2004;34(10):628-637.

52. Cieśla S, Bąk M. The effect of breast reconstruction on maintaining a proper body posture in patients after mastectomy. *Breast Reconstruction—current techniques.* Ed. Marzia Salgarello. http://www.intechopen.com/books/breast-reconstruction-current-techniques/the-influence-of-immediate-breast-reconstruction-on-proper-body-posture-in-women-after-mastectomy-fo

53. Kravitz L, Heyward V. Flexibility Training. http://www.unm.edu/~lkravitz/Article%20folder/flextrain.html.

54. Nelson AG, Kokkonen J, Arnall DA. Twenty minutes of passive stretching lowers glucose levels in an at-risk population: An experimental study. *J Physiother.* 2011;57(3):173-178.

55. Chang RY, Koo M, Ho MY, et al. Effects of Tai Chi on adiponectin and glucose homeostasis in individuals with cardiovascular risk factors. *Eur J Appl Physiol.* Jan 2011;111(1):57-66.

56. Posadzki P, Ernst E. Yoga for low back pain: A systematic review of randomized clinical trials. *Clin Rheumatol.* Sep 2011;30(9):1257-1262.

57. Associated Bodywork & Massage Professionals. Introduction to massage. 2012; http://www.massagetherapy.com/learnmore/index.php. Accessed May 7, 2012.

58. University of Maryland Medical Center. Massage. 2011; http://www.umm.edu/altmed/articles/massage-000354.htm.

59. Labrique-Walusis F, Keister KJ, Russell AC. Massage therapy for stress management: Implications for nursing practice. *Orthop Nurs.* Jul-Aug 2010;29(4):254-257.

60. Rapaport MH, Schettler P, Bresee C. A preliminary study of the effects of a single session of Swedish massage on hypothalamic-pituitary-adrenal and immune function in normal individuals. *J Altern Complement Med.* Sep 1, 2010. Epub.

61. Sajedi F, Kashaninia Z, Hoseinzadeh S, Abedinipoor A. How effective is Swedish massage on blood glucose level in children with diabetes mellitus? *Acta Med Iran.* 2011;49(9):592-597.

Chapter 10

1. Selye H. *The Stress of Life.* Rev. ed. New York: The McGraw-Hill Companies, Inc.; 1976.

2. Chrousos GP. Stress and disorders of the stress system. *Nat Rev Endocrinol.* 2009;5(7):374-381.

3. Pruessner JC, Hellhammer DH, Kirschbaum C. Burnout, perceived stress, and cortisol responses to awakening. *Psychosom Med.* 1999;61(2):197-204.

4. Arafah BM, Nishiyama FJ, Tlaygeh H, Hejal R. Measurement of salivary cortisol concentration in the assessment of adrenal function in critically ill subjects: A surrogate marker of the circulating free cortisol. *J Clin Endocrinol Metab.* 2007;92(8):2965-2971.

5. Starks MA, Starks SL, Kingsley M, Purpura M, Jager R. The effects of phosphatidylserine on endocrine response to moderate intensity exercise. *J Int Soc Sports Nutr.* 2008;5:11.

6. Teh MM, Dunn JT, Choudhary P, et al. Evolution and resolution of human brain perfusion responses to the stress of induced hypoglycemia. *Neuroimage.* Nov 1, 2010;53(2):584-592.

7. Laugero KD, Falcon LM, Tucker KL. Relationship between perceived stress and dietary and activity patterns in older adults participating in the Boston Puerto Rican Health Study. *Appetite.* Feb 2011;56(1):194-204.

8. Dallman MF, Pecoraro N, Akana SF, et al. Chronic stress and obesity: A new view of "comfort food." *Proc Natl Acad Sci U.S.A.* 2003;100(20):11696-11701.

9. Tomiyama AJ, Dallman MF, Epel ES. Comfort food is comforting to those most stressed: Evidence of the chronic stress response network in high stress women. *Psychoneuroendocrinology.* Nov 2011;36(10):1513-1519.

10. Dallman MF, Pecoraro NC, la Fleur SE. Chronic stress and comfort foods: Self-medication and abdominal obesity. *Brain Behav Immun.* 2005;19(4):275-280.

Chapter 11

1. Dunlap Jay CL, Jennifer J., DeCoursey Patricia J., eds. *Chronobiology: Biological Timekeeping.* Sunderland, MA: Sinauer Associates; 2004.

2. Ptitsyn AA, Gimble JM. True or false: All genes are rhythmic. *Ann Med.* Feb 2011;43(1):1-12.

3. Sahar S, Sassone-Corsi P. Regulation of metabolism: The circadian clock dictates the time. *Trends Endocrinol Metab.* Jan 2012;23(1):1-8.

4. Marcheva B, Ramsey KM, Affinati A, Bass J. Clock genes and metabolic disease. *J Appl Physiol.* Nov 2009;107(5):1638-1646.

5. Shaw E, Tofler GH. Circadian rhythm and cardiovascular disease. *Curr Atheroscler Rep.* Jul 2009;11(4):289-295.

6. Janszky I, Ahnve S, Ljung R, et al. Daylight saving time shifts and incidence of acute myocardial infarction--Swedish Register of Information and Knowledge About Swedish Heart Intensive Care Admissions (RIKS-HIA). *Sleep Med.* Mar 2012;13(3):237-242.

7. Alvarez-Saavedra M, Antoun G, Yanagiya A, et al. miRNA-132 orchestrates chromatin remodeling and translational control of the circadian clock. *Hum Mol Genet.* Feb 15 2011;20(4):731-751.

8. Laposky AD, Bass J, Kohsaka A, Turek FW. Sleep and circadian rhythms: Key components in the regulation of energy metabolism. *FEBS Lett.* Jan 9, 2008;582(1):142-151.

9. Patel SR, Hu FB. Short sleep duration and weight gain: A systematic review. *Obesity (Silver Spring).* Mar 2008;16(3):643-653.

10. Knutson KL, Van Cauter E. Associations between sleep loss and increased risk of obesity and diabetes. *Ann N Y Acad Sci.* 2008;1129:287-304.

11. Knutson KL, Spiegel K, Penev P, Van Cauter E. The metabolic consequences of sleep deprivation. *Sleep Med Rev.* Jun 2007;11(3):163-178.

12. Knutson KL. Sleep duration and cardiometabolic risk: A review of the epidemiologic evidence. *Best Pract Res Clin Endocrinol Metab.* Oct 2010;24(5):731-743.

13. Leproult R, Van Cauter E. Role of sleep and sleep loss in hormonal release and metabolism. *Endocr Dev.* 2010;17:11-21.

14. Watson NF, Harden KP, Buchwald D, et al. Sleep duration and body mass index in twins: A gene-environment interaction. *Sleep.* May 1, 2012;35(5):597-603.

15. Elder CR, Gullion CM, Funk KL, Debar LL, Lindberg NM, Stevens VJ. Impact of sleep, screen time, depression and stress on weight change in the intensive weight loss phase of the LIFE study. *International Journal of Obesity (2005).* Jan 2012;36(1):86-92.

16. Nedeltcheva AV, Kilkus JM, Imperial J, Schoeller DA, Penev PD. Insufficient sleep undermines dietary efforts to reduce adiposity. *Ann Intern Med.* Oct 5, 2010;153(7):435-441.

17. Schmid SM, Hallschmid M, Jauch-Chara K, et al. Disturbed glucoregulatory response to food intake after moderate sleep restriction. *Sleep.* Mar 2011;34(3):371-377.

18. Schmid SM, Hallschmid M, Jauch-Chara K, Born J, Schultes B. A single night of sleep deprivation increases ghrelin levels and feelings of hunger in normal-weight healthy men. *J Sleep Res.* Sep 2008;17(3):331-334.

19. Omisade A, Buxton OM, Rusak B. Impact of acute sleep restriction on cortisol and leptin levels in young women. *Physiol Behav.* Apr 19, 2010;99(5):651-656.

20. Kripke DF, Langer RD, Kline LE. Hypnotics' association with mortality or cancer: A matched cohort study. *BMJ Open.* 2012;2(1):e000850.

21. Kegel M, Dam H, Ali F, Bjerregaard P. The prevalence of seasonal affective disorder (SAD) in Greenland is related to latitude. *Nord J Psychiatry.* 2009;63(4):331-335.

22. Mahoney MM. Shift work, jet lag, and female reproduction. *Int J Endocrinol.* 2010;2010:813764.

23. Kott J, Leach G, Yan L. Direction-dependent effects of chronic "jet-lag" on hippocampal neurogenesis. *Neurosci Lett.* May 2, 2012;515(2):177-180.

24. Szosland D. Shift work and metabolic syndrome, diabetes mellitus and ischaemic heart disease. *Int J Occup Med Environ Health.* 2010;23(3):287-291.

25. Esquirol Y, Bongard V, Mabile L, Jonnier B, Soulat JM, Perret B. Shift work and metabolic syndrome: Respective impacts of job strain, physical activity, and dietary rhythms. *Chronobiol Int.* Apr 2009;26(3):544-559.

26. Lin YC, Hsiao TJ, Chen PC. Persistent rotating shift-work exposure accelerates development of metabolic syndrome among middle-aged female employees: A five-year follow-up. *Chronobiol Int.* May 2009;26(4):740-755.

27. Antunes LC, Levandovski R, Dantas G, Caumo W, Hidalgo MP. Obesity and shift work: Chronobiological aspects. *Nutrition Research Reviews.* Jun 2010;23(1):155-168.

28. Yan L. Structural and functional changes in the suprachiasmatic nucleus following chronic circadian rhythm perturbation. *Neuroscience.* Jun 2, 2011;183:99-107.

29. Puttonen S, Viitasalo K, Harma M. The relationship between current and former shift work and the metabolic syndrome. *Scand J Work Environ Health.* Jan 9, 2012;pii:3267. Epub.

30. Pan A, Schernhammer ES, Sun Q, Hu FB. Rotating night shift work and risk of type 2 diabetes: Two prospective cohort studies in women. *PLoS Med.* Dec 2011;8(12): e1001141.

31. Biggi N, Consonni D, Galluzzo V, Sogliani M, Costa G. Metabolic syndrome in permanent night workers. *Chronobiol Int.* Apr 2008;25(2):443-454.

32. Pimenta AM, Kac G, Souza RR, Ferreira LM, Silqueira SM. Night-shift work and cardiovascular risk among employees of a public university. *Rev Assoc Med Bras.* Apr 2012;58(2):168-177.

33. Sasseville A, Benhaberou-Brun D, Fontaine C, Charon MC, Hebert M. Wearing blue-blockers in the morning could improve sleep of workers on a permanent night schedule: A pilot study. *Chronobiol Int.* Jul 2009;26(5):913-925.

34. Milner CE, Cote KA. Benefits of napping in healthy adults: Impact of nap length, time of day, age, and experience with napping. *J Sleep Res.* Jun 2009;18(2):272-281.

35. Dhand R, Sohal H. Good sleep, bad sleep! The role of daytime naps in healthy adults. *Curr Opin Pulm Med.* Nov 2006;12(6):379-382.

36. Warner S, Murray G, Meyer D. Holiday and school-term sleep patterns of Australian adolescents. *J Adolesc.* Oct 2008;31(5):595-608.

37. Wing YK, Li SX, Li AM, Zhang J, Kong AP. The effect of weekend and holiday sleep compensation on childhood overweight and obesity. *Pediatrics.* Nov 2009;124(5):e994-e1000.

38. Hazlerigg DG, Lincoln GA. Hypothesis: Cyclical histogenesis is the basis of circannual timing. *J Biol Rhythms.* Dec 2011;26(6):471-485.

39. Lincoln GA, Hazlerigg DG. Mammalian circannual pacemakers. *Soc Reprod Fertil Suppl.* 2010;67:171-186.

40. Cizza G, Requena M, Galli G, de Jonge L. Chronic sleep deprivation and seasonality: Implications for the obesity epidemic. *J Endocrinol Invest.* Nov 2011;34(10):793-800.

41. Stress TAIo. Job stress. http://www.stress.org/job.htm. Accessed April 24, 2012.

42. Dickler J. Americans to forfeit $34.3 billion in vacation days. 2011; http://money.cnn.com/2011/11/30/pf/unused_vacation/index.htm. Accessed April 24, 2012.

43. Expedia.com. Vacation deprivation by country. : http://www.expedia.com/p/info-other/vacation_deprivation.htm. Accessed April 24, 2012.

44. Levi F, Halberg F. Circaseptan (about-7-day) bioperiodicity--spontaneous and reactive--and the search for pacemakers. *Ric Clin Lab.* Apr-Jun 1982;12(2):323-370.

45. Otsuka K, Yamanaka G, Shinagawa M, et al. Chronomic community screening reveals about 31% depression, elevated blood pressure and infradian vascular rhythm alteration. *Biomed Pharmacother.* Oct 2004;58 Suppl 1:S48-55.

46. Lee MS, Lee JS, Lee JY, Cornelissen G, Otsuka K, Halberg F. About 7-day (circaseptan) and circadian changes in cold pressor test (CPT). *Biomed Pharmacother.* Oct 2003;57 Suppl 1:39S-44S.

47. Witte DR, Grobbee DE, Bots ML, Hoes AW. Excess cardiac mortality on Monday: The importance of gender, age and hospitalisation. *Eur J Epidemiol.* 2005;20(5):395-399.

48. Besarab A, Wesson L, Jarrell B, Burke JF. Effect of delayed graft function and ALG on the circaseptan (about 7-day) rhythm of human renal allograft rejection. *Transplantation.* Jun 1983;35(6):562-566.

49. Guan J, You C, Liu Y, Zhang R, Wang Z. Characteristics of infradian and circadian rhythms in the persistent vegetative state. *J Int Med Res.* 2011;39(6):2281-2287.

50. Cornelissen G, Halberg F, Breus TK, et al. [The origin of the biological week from data on the rhythm of cardiac contractions in people during the solar activity cycle]. *Biofizika.* Jul-Aug 1998;43(4):666-669.

51. Aron C. The history of the vacation examined. 2009. http://www.npr.org/templates/story/story.php?storyId=105545388. Accessed April 24, 2012.

52. Chikani V, Reding D, Gunderson P, McCarty CA. Vacations improve mental health among rural women: The Wisconsin Rural Women's Health Study. *WMJ*. Aug 2005;104(6):20-23.

53. Gump BB, Matthews KA. Are vacations good for your health? The 9-year mortality experience after the multiple risk factor intervention trial. *Psychosom Med*. Sep-Oct 2000;62(5):608-612.

54. Strauss-Blasche G, Reithofer B, Schobersberger W, Ekmekcioglu C, Marktl W. Effect of vacation on health: Moderating factors of vacation outcome. *J Travel Med*. Mar-Apr 2005;12(2):94-101.

55. Strauss-Blasche G, Ekmekcioglu C, Marktl W. Does vacation enable recuperation? Changes in well-being associated with time away from work. *Occup Med (Lond)*. Apr 2000;50(3):167-172.

56. De Bloom J, Geurts SA, Sonnentag S, Taris T, de Weerth C, Kompier MA. How does a vacation from work affect employee health and well-being? *Psychol Health*. Dec 2011;26(12):1606-1622.

57. Fritz C, Sonnentag S. Recovery, well-being, and performance-related outcomes: The role of workload and vacation experiences. *J Appl Psychol*. Jul 2006;91(4):936-945.

Chapter 12

1. Holick MF. Vitamin D: Extraskeletal health. *Endocrinol Metab Clin North Am*. Jun 2010;39(2):381-400, table of contents.

2. Holick MF. Vitamin D: Extraskeletal health. *Rheum Dis Clin North Am*. Feb 2012;38(1):141-160.

3. Hagenau T, Vest R, Gissel TN, et al. Global vitamin D levels in relation to age, gender, skin pigmentation and latitude: An ecologic meta-regression analysis. *Osteoporos Int*. Jan 2009;20(1):133-140.

4. IOM. Dietary reference intakes for calcium and vitamin D. 2010; http://www.iom.edu/Reports/2010/Dietary-Reference-Intakes-for-Calcium-and-Vitamin-D.aspx. Accessed May 31, 2012.

5. Lioy PJ, Rappaport SM. Exposure science and the exposome: An opportunity for coherence in the environmental health sciences. *Environmental Health Perspectives*. Nov 2011;119(11):A466-467.

6. Rappaport SM. Discovering environmental causes of disease. *J Epidemiol Community Health*. Feb 2012;66(2):99-102.

7. Vom Saal FS, Nagel SC, Coe BL, Angle BM, Taylor JA. The estrogenic endocrine disrupting chemical bisphenol A (BPA) and obesity. *Mol Cell Endocrinol*. May 6, 2012;354(1-2):74-84.

8. Schug TT, Janesick A, Blumberg B, Heindel JJ. Endocrine disrupting chemicals and disease susceptibility. *J Steroid Biochem Mol Biol*. Nov 2011;127(3-5):204-215.

9. Beronius A, Ruden C, Hakansson H, Hanberg A. Risk to all or none? A comparative analysis of controversies in the health risk assessment of Bisphenol A. *Reprod Toxicol.* Apr 2010;29(2):132-146.

10. Shankar A, Teppala S. Urinary bisphenol A and hypertension in a multiethnic sample of US adults. *J Environ Public Health.* 2012;2012:481641.

11. Melzer D, Osborne NJ, Henley WE, et al. Urinary bisphenol A concentration and risk of future coronary artery disease in apparently healthy men and women. *Circulation.* Mar 27, 2012;125(12):1482-1490.

12. Shankar A, Teppala S. Relationship between urinary bisphenol A levels and diabetes mellitus. *J Clin Endocrinol Metab.* Dec 2011;96(12):3822-3826.

13. Meeker JD. Exposure to environmental endocrine disrupting compounds and men's health. *Maturitas.* Jul 2010;66(3):236-241.

14. Kundakovic M, Champagne FA. Epigenetic perspective on the developmental effects of bisphenol A. *Brain Behav Immun.* Aug 2011;25(6):1084-1093.

15. Weng YI, Hsu PY, Liyanarachchi S, et al. Epigenetic influences of low-dose bisphenol A in primary human breast epithelial cells. *Toxicol Appl Pharmacol.* Oct 15, 2010;248(2):111-121.

16. Dolinoy DC, Huang D, Jirtle RL. Maternal nutrient supplementation counteracts bisphenol A-induced DNA hypomethylation in early development. *Proc Natl Acad Sci U S A.* Aug 7, 2007;104(32):13056-13061.

17. Jaakkola JJ, Knight TL. The role of exposure to phthalates from polyvinyl chloride products in the development of asthma and allergies: A systematic review and meta-analysis. *Environmental Health Perspectives.* Jul 2008;116(7):845-853.

18. Svechnikov K, Izzo G, Landreh L, Weisser J, Soder O. Endocrine disruptors and Leydig cell function. *J Biomed Biotechnol.* 2010;2010.

19. Stahlhut RW, van Wijngaarden E, Dye TD, Cook S, Swan SH. Concentrations of urinary phthalate metabolites are associated with increased waist circumference and insulin resistance in adult U.S. males. *Environmental Health Perspectives.* Jun 2007;115(6):876-882.

20. Lind PM, Roos V, Ronn M, et al. Serum concentrations of phthalate metabolites related to abdominal fat distribution two years later in elderly women. *Environ Health.* Apr 2, 2012;11(1):21.

21. WHO. Dioxins and their effect on human health. 2010; http://www.who.int/mediacentre/factsheets/fs225/en/.

22. Bradshaw TD, Bell DR. Relevance of the aryl hydrocarbon receptor (AhR) for clinical toxicology. *Clin Toxicol (Phila).* Aug 2009;47(7):632-642.

23. Ishida T, Takeda T, Koga T, et al. Attenuation of 2,3,7,8-tetrachlorodibenzo-p-dioxin toxicity by resveratrol: A comparative study with different routes of administration. *Biol Pharm Bull.* May 2009;32(5):876-881.

24. Degner SC, Papoutsis AJ, Selmin O, Romagnolo DF. Targeting of aryl hydrocarbon receptor-mediated activation of cyclooxygenase-2 expression by the indole-3-carbinol metabolite 3,3'-diindolylmethane in breast cancer cells. *J Nutr.* Jan 2009;139(1):26-32.

25. Geier DA, King PG, Sykes LK, Geier MR. A comprehensive review of mercury provoked autism. *Indian J Med Res.* Oct 2008;128(4):383-411.

26. Houston MC. Role of mercury toxicity in hypertension, cardiovascular disease, and stroke. *J Clin Hypertens (Greenwich).* Aug 2011;13(8):621-627.

27. Guallar E, Sanz-Gallardo MI, van't Veer P, et al. Mercury, fish oils, and the risk of myocardial infarction. *N Engl J Med.* Nov 28, 2002;347(22):1747-1754.

28. Boffetta P, Sallsten G, Garcia-Gomez M, et al. Mortality from cardiovascular diseases and exposure to inorganic mercury. *Occup Environ Med.* Jul 2001;58(7):461-466.

29. Crespo-Lopez ME, Macedo GL, Pereira SI, et al. Mercury and human genotoxicity: Critical considerations and possible molecular mechanisms. *Pharmacol Res.* Oct 2009;60(4):212-220.

30. Falluel-Morel A, Lin L, Sokolowski K, McCandlish E, Buckley B, DiCicco-Bloom E. N-acetyl cysteine treatment reduces mercury-induced neurotoxicity in the developing rat hippocampus. *J Neurosci Res.* Apr 2012;90(4):743-750.

31. Anuradha B, Varalakshmi P. Protective role of DL-alpha-lipoic acid against mercury-induced neural lipid peroxidation. *Pharmacol Res.* Jan 1999;39(1):67-80.

32. Deng Y, Xu Z, Liu W, Yang H, Xu B, Wei Y. Effects of lycopene and proanthocyanidins on hepatotoxicity induced by mercuric chloride in rats. *Biol Trace Elem Res.* May 2012;146(2):213-223.

33. Liu W, Xu Z, Yang H, Deng Y, Xu B, Wei Y. The protective effects of tea polyphenols and schisandrin B on nephrotoxicity of mercury. *Biol Trace Elem Res.* Dec 2011;143(3):1651-1665.

34. Barcelos GR, Angeli JP, Serpeloni JM, et al. Quercetin protects human-derived liver cells against mercury-induced DNA-damage and alterations of the redox status. *Mutat Res.* Dec 24, 2011;726(2):109-115.

35. El-Shenawy SM, Hassan NS. Comparative evaluation of the protective effect of selenium and garlic against liver and kidney damage induced by mercury chloride in the rats. *Pharmacol Rep.* Mar-Apr 2008;60(2):199-208.

36. Abdalla FH, Belle LP, De Bona KS, Bitencourt PE, Pigatto AS, Moretto MB. Allium sativum L. extract prevents methyl mercury-induced cytotoxicity in peripheral blood leukocytes (LS). *Food and chemical toxicology: An international journal published for the British Industrial Biological Research Association.* Jan 2010;48(1):417-421.

37. Joshi D, Mittal D, Shrivastav S, Shukla S, Srivastav AK. Combined effect of N-acetyl cysteine, zinc, and selenium against chronic dimethylmercury-induced oxidative stress: A biochemical and histopathological approach. *Archives of Environmental Contamination and Toxicology.* Nov 2011;61(4):558-567.

38. CDC. Lead-Prevention Tips. 2009; http://www.cdc.gov/nceh/lead/tips.htm.

39. Nemsadze K, Sanikidze T, Ratiani L, Gabunia L, Sharashenidze T. Mechanisms of lead-induced poisoning. *Georgian Med News.* Jul-Aug 2009(172-173):92-96.

40. Vaziri ND. Mechanisms of lead-induced hypertension and cardiovascular disease. *Am J Physiol Heart Circ Physiol.* Aug 2008;295(2):H454-465.

41. Hsu PC, Guo YL. Antioxidant nutrients and lead toxicity. *Toxicology.* Oct 30, 2002;180(1):33-44.

42. Patrick L. Lead toxicity part II: The role of free radical damage and the use of antioxidants in the pathology and treatment of lead toxicity. *Altern Med Rev.* Jun 2006;11(2):114-127.

43. Prins GS. Endocrine disruptors and prostate cancer risk. *Endocr Relat Cancer.* 2008;15:649-656.

44. Jomova K, Jenisova Z, Feszterova M, et al. Arsenic: Toxicity, oxidative stress and human disease. *J Appl Toxicol.* Mar 2011;31(2):95-107.

45. Rossman TG. Mechanism of arsenic carcinogenesis: An integrated approach. *Mutat Res.* Dec 10, 2003;533(1-2):37-65.

46. Navas-Acien A, Silbergeld EK, Pastor-Barriuso R, Guallar E. Arsenic exposure and prevalence of type 2 diabetes in US adults. *JAMA.* Aug 20, 2008;300(7):814-822.

47. Celik I, Gallicchio L, Boyd K, et al. Arsenic in drinking water and lung cancer: A systematic review. *Environ Res.* Sep 2008;108(1):48-55.

48. Tomljenovic L. Aluminum and Alzheimer's disease: After a century of controversy, is there a plausible link? *Journal of Alzheimer's Disease: JAD.* 2011;23(4):567-598.

49. Rondeau V, Jacqmin-Gadda H, Commenges D, Helmer C, Dartigues JF. Aluminum and silica in drinking water and the risk of Alzheimer's disease or cognitive decline: Findings from 15-year follow-up of the PAQUID cohort. *Am J Epidemiol.* 2009;169:489-496.

50. Yumoto S, Kakimi S, Ohsaki A, Ishikawa A. Demonstration of aluminum in amyloid fibers in the cores of senile plaques in the brains of patients with Alzheimer's disease. *J Inorg Biochem.* 2009;103:1579-1584.

51. McLachlan DR, Bergeron C, Smith JE, Boomer D, Rifat SL. Risk for neuropathologically confirmed Alzheimer's disease and residual aluminum in municipal drinking water employing weighted residential histories. *Neurology.* Feb 1996;46(2):401-405.

52. Exley C, Charles LM, Barr L, Martin C, Polwart A, Darbre PD. Aluminum in human breast tissue. *J Inorg Biochem.* 2007;101:1344-1346.

53. Ferreira PC, Piai Kde A, Takayanagui AM, Segura-Munoz SI. Aluminum as a risk factor for Alzheimer's disease. *Rev Lat Am Enfermagem.* 2008;16:151-157.

54. Crinnion WJ. Environmental medicine, part 4: Pesticides—biologically persistent and ubiquitous toxins. *Altern Med Rev.* Oct 2000;5(5):432-447.

55. Kuhnlein HV, Receveur O, Muir DC, Chan HM, Soueida R. Arctic indigenous women consume greater than acceptable levels of organochlorines. *J Nutr.* Oct 1995;125(10):2501-2510.

56. Jensen GE, Clausen J. Organochlorine compounds in adipose tissue of Greenlanders and southern Danes. *Journal of Toxicology and Environmental Health.* Jul 1979;5(4):617-629.

57. Archibeque-Engle SL, Tessari JD, Winn DT, Keefe TJ, Nett TM, Zheng T. Comparison of organochlorine pesticide and polychlorinated biphenyl residues in human breast adipose tissue and serum. *Journal of Toxicology and Environmental Health.* Nov 1997;52(4):285-293.

58. Inmaculada Sanz-Gallardo M, Guallar E, van Tveer P, et al. Determinants of p,p-dichlorodiphenyldichloroethane (DDE) concentration in adipose tissue in women from five European cities. *Archives of environmental health.* Jul-Aug 1999;54(4):277-283.

59. Ben-Michael E, Grauer F, Raphael C, Sahm Z, Richter ED. Organochlorine insecticides and PCB residues in fat tissues of autopsied trauma victims in Israel: 1984 to 1986. *Journal of Environmental Pathology, Toxicology and Oncology: Official Organ of the International Society for Environmental Toxicology and Cancer.* 1999;18(4):297-303.

60. Van der Ven K, van der Ven H, Thibold A, et al. Chlorinated hydrocarbon content of fetal and maternal body tissues and fluids in full term pregnant women: A comparison of Germany versus Tanzania. *Human Reproduction (Oxford, England).* Jun 1992;7 Suppl 1:95-100.

61. Llop S, Ballester F, Vizcaino E, et al. Concentrations and determinants of organochlorine levels among pregnant women in Eastern Spain. *Sci Total Environ.* 2010; 408:5758-5767.

62. Sagiv SK, Thurston SW, Bellinger DC, Tolbert PE, Altshul LM, Korrick SA. Prenatal organochlorine exposure and behaviors associated with attention deficit hyperactivity disorder in school-aged children. *Am J Epidemiol.* 2010;171:593-601.

63. Kanja LW, Skaare JU, Ojwang SB, Maitai CK. A comparison of organochlorine pesticide residues in maternal adipose tissue, maternal blood, cord blood, and human milk from mother/infant pairs. *Archives of Environmental Contamination and Toxicology.* Jan 1992;22(1):21-24.

64. Frank R, Rasper J, Smout MS, Braun HE. Organochlorine residues in adipose tissues, blood and milk from Ontario residents, 1976-1985. *Canadian Journal of Public Health. Revue canadienne de sante publique.* May-Jun 1988;79(3):150-158.

65. Lensen G, Jungbauer F, Goncalo M, Coenraads PJ. Airborne irritant contact dermatitis and conjunctivitis after occupational exposure to chlorothalonil in textiles. *Contact Dermatitis.* 2007;57:181-186.

66. Sharma SK, Tyagi PK, Upadhyay AK, et al. Efficacy of permethrin treated long-lasting insecticidal nets on malaria transmission and observations on the perceived side effects, collateral benefits and human safety in a hyperendemic tribal area of Orissa, India. *Acta Trop.* Nov 2009;112(2):181-187.

67. Adams RD, Lupton D, Good AM, Bateman DN. UK childhood exposures to pesticides 2004-2007: A TOXBASE toxicovigilance study. *Arch Dis Child.* Jun 2009;94(6):417-420.

68. Casals-Casas C, Desvergne B. Endocrine disruptors: From endocrine to metabolic disruption. *Annual Review of Physiology.* Mar 17, 2011;73:135-162.

69. Stefanidou M, Maravelias C, Spiliopoulou C. Human exposure to endocrine disruptors and breast milk. *Endocr Metab Immune Disord Drug Targets.* 2009;9:269-276.

70. Dishaw LV, Powers CM, Ryde IT, et al. Is the PentaBDE replacement, tris (1,3-dichloro-2-propyl) phosphate (TDCPP), a developmental neurotoxicant? Studies in PC12 cells. *Toxicol Appl Pharmacol.* 2011;256(3):281-289.

71. Franco R, Li S, Rodriguez-Rocha H, Burns M, Panayiotidis MI. Molecular mechanisms of pesticide-induced neurotoxicity: Relevance to Parkinson's disease. *Chem Biol Interact.* 2010;188:289-300.

72. Wassermann M, Nogueira DP, Tomatis L, et al. Organochlorine compounds in neoplastic and adjacent apparently normal breast tissue. *Bulletin of Environmental Contamination and Toxicology.* Apr 1976;15(4):478-484.

73. Mussalo-Rauhamaa H, Hasanen E, Pyysalo H, Antervo K, Kauppila R, Pantzar P. Occurrence of beta-hexachlorocyclohexane in breast cancer patients. *Cancer.* Nov 15, 1990;66(10):2124-2128.

74. Falck F, Jr., Ricci A, Jr., Wolff MS, Godbold J, Deckers P. Pesticides and polychlorinated biphenyl residues in human breast lipids and their relation to breast cancer. *Archives of Environmental Health.* Mar-Apr 1992;47(2):143-146.

75. Rundle A, Hoepner L, Hassoun A, et al. Association of childhood obesity with maternal exposure to ambient air polycyclic aromatic hydrocarbons during pregnancy. *Am J Epidemiol.* Apr 13, 2012;175(11):1163-72.

76. Bassil KL, Vakil C, Sanborn M, Cole DC, Kaur JS, Kerr KJ. Cancer health effects of pesticides: Systematic review. *Can Fam Physician.* 2007;53:1704-1711.

77. Yiee JH, Baskin LS. Environmental factors in genitourinary development. *J Urol.* 2010;184:34-41.

78. Giordano F, Abballe A, De Felip E, et al. Maternal exposures to endocrine disrupting chemicals and hypospadias in offspring. *Birth Defects Research. Part A, Clinical and Molecular Teratology.* Apr 2010;88(4):241-250.

79. Sanborn M, Kerr KJ, Sanin LH, Cole DC, Bassil KL, Vakil C. Non-cancer health effects of pesticides: Systematic review and implications for family doctors. *Can Fam Physician.* 2007;53:1712-1720.

80. Jurewicz J, Hanke W. Prenatal and childhood exposure to pesticides and neurobehavioral development: Review of epidemiological studies. *Int J Occup Med Environ Health.* 2008;21:121-132.

81. De Vocht F. "Dirty electricity": What, where, and should we care? *J Expo Sci Environ Epidemiol.* Jul 2010;20(5):399-405.

82. Bioinitiative. BioInitiative Report: A Rationale for a Biologically-based Public Exposure Standard for Electromagnetic Fields (ELF and RF). http://www.bioinitiative.org/freeaccess/report/index.htm.

83. Abraham A, Sommerhalder K, Abel T. Landscape and well-being: A scoping study on the health-promoting impact of outdoor environments. *Int J Public Health.* Feb 2010;55(1):59-69.

84. Depledge MH, Stone RJ, Bird WJ. Can natural and virtual environments be used to promote improved human health and wellbeing? *Environ Sci Technol.* Jun 1, 2011;45(11):4660-4665.

85. Riediker M, Koren HS. The importance of environmental exposures to physical, mental and social well-being. *Int J Hyg Environ Health.* Jul 2004;207(3):193-201.

86. Chevalier G, Sinatra ST, Oschman JL, Sokal K, Sokal P. Earthing: Health implications of reconnecting the human body to the Earth's surface electrons. *J Environ Public Health.* 2012;2012:291541.

87. Ghaly M, Teplitz D. The biologic effects of grounding the human body during sleep as measured by cortisol levels and subjective reporting of sleep, pain, and stress. *J Altern Complement Med.* Oct 2004;10(5):767-776.

88. Sokal K, Sokal P. Earthing the human body influences physiologic processes. *J Altern Complement Med.* Apr 2011;17(4):301-308.

89. Loomba RS, Arora R, Shah PH, Chandrasekar S, Molnar J. Effects of music on systolic blood pressure, diastolic blood pressure, and heart rate: A meta-analysis. *Indian Heart J.* May-Jun 2012;64(3):309-313.

90. Trappe HJ. The effects of music on the cardiovascular system and cardiovascular health. *Heart.* Dec 2010;96(23):1868-1871.

91. Young VB. The intestinal microbiota in health and disease. *Curr Opin Gastroenterol.* Jan 2012;28(1):63-69.

92. Stewardson AJ, Huttner B, Harbarth S. At least it won't hurt: The personal risks of antibiotic exposure. *Curr Opin Pharmacol.* Oct 2011;11(5):446-452.

93. Vaishnavi C. Clostridium difficile infection: Clinical spectrum and approach to management. *Indian J Gastroenterol.* Dec 2011;30(6):245-254.

94. Kaplan JL, Shi HN, Walker WA. The role of microbes in developmental immunologic programming. *Pediatr Res.* Jun 2011;69(6):465-472.

95. Hempel S, Newberry SJ, Maher AR, et al. Probiotics for the prevention and treatment of antibiotic-associated diarrhea: A systematic review and meta-analysis. *JAMA.* May 9, 2012;307(18):1959-1969.

96. Johnston BC, Goldenberg JZ, Vandvik PO, Sun X, Guyatt GH. Probiotics for the prevention of pediatric antibiotic-associated diarrhea. *Cochrane Database Syst Rev.* 2011(11):CD004827.

97. Aureli P, Capurso L, Castellazzi AM, et al. Probiotics and health: An evidence-based review. *Pharmacol Res.* May 2011;63(5):366-376.

Chapter 13

1. Aiello AE, Larson EL, Levy SB. Consumer antibacterial soaps: Effective or just risky? *Clin Infect Dis.* Sep 1, 2007;45 Suppl 2:S137-147.

2. Frei R, Lauener RP, Crameri R, O'Mahony L. Microbiota and dietary interactions: An update to the hygiene hypothesis? *Allergy.* Apr 2012;67(4):451-461.

3. Fishbein AB, Fuleihan RL. The hygiene hypothesis revisited: Does exposure to infectious agents protect us from allergy? *Curr Opin Pediatr.* Feb 2012;24(1):98-102.

4. Ngoi SM, Sylvester FA, Vella AT. The role of microbial byproducts in protection against immunological disorders and the hygiene hypothesis. *Discov Med.* Nov 2011;12(66):405-412.

5. Bach JF, Chatenoud L. The hygiene hypothesis: An explanation for the increased frequency of insulin-dependent diabetes. *Cold Spring Harb Perspect Med.* Feb 2012;2(2): a007799.

6. Edwards J. 2012; http://ultimatewestu.com/stories/338668-survey-finds-12-percent-of-americans-practice-healthy-habits.

7. Koren O, Spor A, Felin J, et al. Human oral, gut, and plaque microbiota in patients with atherosclerosis. *Proc Natl Acad Sci U S A*. 2011;1:4592-4598.

8. Zeigler CC, Persson GR, Wondimu B, Marcus C, Sobko T, Modeer T. Microbiota in the oral subgingival biofilm is associated with obesity in adolescence. *Obesity (Silver Spring)*. Jan 2012;20(1):157-164.

9. Goodson JM, Groppo D, Halem S, Carpino E. Is obesity an oral bacterial disease? *J Dent Res*. Jun 2009;88(6):519-523.

10. Clarke S, Murphy E, Nilaweera K, et al. The gut microbiota and its relationship to diet and obesity: New insights. *Gut Microbes*. May 1, 2012;3(3).

11. Avila M, Ojcius DM, Yilmaz O. The oral microbiota: Living with a permanent guest. *DNA Cell Biol*. Aug 2009;28(8):405-411.

12. Zarco MF, Vess TJ, Ginsburg GS. The oral microbiome in health and disease and the potential impact on personalized dental medicine. *Oral Dis*. Mar 2012;18(2):109-120.

13. CDC. Smoking and Tobacco Use - Fast Facts. http://www.cdc.gov/tobacco/data_statistics/fact_sheets/fast_facts/index.htm. Accessed May 8, 2012.

14. Tanne JH. Teenage smoking is an "epidemic," says US surgeon general. *BMJ*. 2012;344:e2004.

15. Brody JS, Steiling K. Interaction of cigarette exposure and airway epithelial cell gene expression. *Annual Review of Physiology*. 2011;73:437-456.

16. Rajendrasozhan S, Yang SR, Edirisinghe I, Yao H, Adenuga D, Rahman I. Deacetylases and NF-kappaB in redox regulation of cigarette smoke-induced lung inflammation: Epigenetics in pathogenesis of COPD. *Antioxid Redox Signal*. Apr 2008;10(4):799-811.

17. Maccani MA, Knopik VS. Cigarette smoke exposure-associated alterations to non-coding RNA. *Front Genet*. 2012;3:53.

18. Volkow ND. Epigenetics of nicotine: Another nail in the coughing. *Sci Transl Med*. Nov 2, 2011;3(107):107ps43.

19. CDC. Alcohol Use and Health - Fact Sheet. http://www.cdc.gov/alcohol/fact-sheets/alcohol-use.htm. Accessed May 8, 2012.

20. Romeo J, Warnberg J, Nova E, Diaz LE, Gomez-Martinez S, Marcos A. Moderate alcohol consumption and the immune system: A review. *The British Journal of Nutrition*. Oct 2007;98 Suppl 1:S111-S115.

21. Eidelman RS, Vignola P, Hennekens CH. Alcohol consumption and coronary heart disease: A causal and protective factor. *Semin Vasc Med*. Aug 2002;2(3):253-256.

22. Cleophas TJ. Wine, beer and spirits and the risk of myocardial infarction: A systematic review. *Biomed Pharmacother*. Oct 1999;53(9):417-423.

23. Zhou FC, Balaraman Y, Teng M, Liu Y, Singh RP, Nephew KP. Alcohol alters DNA methylation patterns and inhibits neural stem cell differentiation. *Alcohol Clin Exp Res*. Apr 2011;35(4):735-746.

24. Kovatsi L, Fragou D, Samanidou V, Njau S, Kouidou S. Drugs of abuse: Epigenetic mechanisms in toxicity and addiction. *Curr Med Chem*. 2011;18(12):1765-1774.

25. MacArthur AC, McBride ML, Spinelli JJ, Tamaro S, Gallagher RP, Theriault G. Risk of childhood leukemia associated with parental smoking and alcohol consumption prior to conception and during pregnancy: The cross-Canada childhood leukemia study. *Cancer Causes Control.* Apr 2008;19(3):283-295.

26. Wong CC, Mill J, Fernandes C. Drugs and addiction: An introduction to epigenetics. *Addiction.* Mar 2011;106(3):480-489.

27. Maze I, Nestler EJ. The epigenetic landscape of addiction. *Ann N Y Acad Sci.* Jan 2011;1216:99-113.

28. CDC. STD Trends in the United States: 2010 National Data for Gonorrhea, Chlamydia, and Syphilis. 2011; http://www.cdc.gov/std/stats10/trends.htm. Accessed May 21, 2012.

29. Joffe GP, Foxman B, Schmidt AJ, et al. Multiple partners and partner choice as risk factors for sexually transmitted disease among female college students. *Sex Transm Dis.* Sep-Oct 1992;19(5):272-278.

30. Fethers KA, Fairley CK, Hocking JS, Gurrin LC, Bradshaw CS. Sexual risk factors and bacterial vaginosis: A systematic review and meta-analysis. *Clin Infect Dis.* Dec 1, 2008;47(11):1426-1435.

31. Chen L, Jha P, Stirling B, et al. Sexual risk factors for HIV infection in early and advanced HIV epidemics in sub-Saharan Africa: Systematic overview of 68 epidemiological studies. *PloS one.* 2007;2(10):e1001.

32. Patavino GM, de Almeida-Neto C, Liu J, et al. Number of recent sexual partners among blood donors in Brazil: Associations with donor demographics, donation characteristics, and infectious disease markers. *Transfusion.* Jan 2012;52(1):151-159.

33. Van Wagoner NJ, Harbison HS, Drewry J, Turnipseed E, Hook EW, III. Characteristics of women reporting multiple recent sex partners presenting to a sexually transmitted disease clinic for care. *Sex Transm Dis.* Mar 2011;38(3):210-215.

34. Cooper ML. Alcohol use and risky sexual behavior among college students and youth: Evaluating the evidence. *J Stud Alcohol Suppl.* Mar 2002(14):101-117.

35. Patel AL, Chaudhry U, Sachdev D, Sachdeva PN, Bala M, Saluja D. An insight into the drug resistance profile & mechanism of drug resistance in Neisseria gonorrhoeae. *Indian J Med Res.* Oct 2011;134:419-431.

36. CDC. Sexually Transmitted Diseases in the United States, 2008. 2009; http://www.cdc. gov/std/stats08/trends.htm. Accessed May 21, 2012.

Chapter 14

1. Dawkins R. *The Blind Watchmaker: Why the Evidence of Evolution Reveals a Universe without Design.* New York: W.W. Norton & Company, Inc; 1996.

2. Boyle PA, Buchman AS, Wilson RS, Yu L, Schneider JA, Bennett DA. Effect of purpose in life on the relation between Alzheimer disease pathologic changes on cognitive function in advanced age. *Arch Gen Psychiatry.* May 2012;69(5):499-504.

3. Toussaint LL, Owen AD, Cheadle A. Forgive to live: Forgiveness, health, and longevity. *J Behav Med.* Jun 25, 2011;35(4):375-86.

4. Hummer RA, Rogers RG, Nam CB, Ellison CG. Religious involvement and U.S. adult mortality. *Demography.* May 1999;36(2):273-285.

5. Hummer RA, Ellison CG, Rogers RG, Moulton BE, Romero RR. Religious involvement and adult mortality in the United States: Review and perspective. *South Med J.* Dec 2004;97(12):1223-1230.

6. Rendall MS, Weden MM, Favreault MM, Waldron H. The protective effect of marriage for survival: A review and update. *Demography.* May 2011;48(2):481-506.

7. Tomcikova Z, Madarasova Geckova A, Orosova O, van Dijk JP, Reijneveld SA. Parental divorce and adolescent drunkenness: Role of socioeconomic position, psychological well-being and social support. *Eur Addict Res.* 2009;15(4):202-208.

8. Huurre T, Lintonen T, Kaprio J, Pelkonen M, Marttunen M, Aro H. Adolescent risk factors for excessive alcohol use at age 32 years. A 16-year prospective follow-up study. *Soc Psychiatry Psychiatr Epidemiol.* Jan 2010;45(1):125-134.

9. Thompson RG, Jr., Lizardi D, Keyes KM, Hasin DS. Childhood or adolescent parental divorce/separation, parental history of alcohol problems, and offspring lifetime alcohol dependence. *Drug Alcohol Depend.* Dec 1, 2008;98(3):264-269.

10. Tomcikova Z, Madarasova Geckova A, Reijneveld SA, van Dijk JP. Parental divorce, adolescents' feelings toward parents and drunkenness in adolescents. *Eur Addict Res.* 2011;17(3):113-118.

11. Van den Eijnden RJ, Meerkerk GJ, Vermulst AA, Spijkerman R, Engels RC. Online communication, compulsive Internet use, and psychosocial well-being among adolescents: A longitudinal study. *Dev Psychol.* May 2008;44(3):655-665.

12. Kraut R, Patterson M, Lundmark V, Kiesler S, Mukopadhyay T, Scherlis W. Internet paradox. A social technology that reduces social involvement and psychological well-being? *Am Psychol.* Sep 1998;53(9):1017-1031.

13. Subrahmanyam K, Lin G. Adolescents on the net: Internet use and well-being. *Adolescence.* Winter 2007;42(168):659-677.

14. Minniti A, Bissoli L, Di Francesco V, et al. Individual versus group therapy for obesity: Comparison of dropout rate and treatment outcome. *Eat Weight Disord.* Dec 2007;12(4):161-167.

15. Feng CY, Chu H, Chen CH, et al. The effect of cognitive behavioral group therapy for depression: A meta-analysis 2000-2010. *Worldviews Evid Based Nurs.* Feb 2012;9(1):2-17.

16. Wild B, Herzog W, Wesche D, Niehoff D, Muller B, Hain B. Development of a group therapy to enhance treatment motivation and decision making in severely obese patients with a comorbid mental disorder. *Obes Surg.* May 2011;21(5):588-594.

INDEX

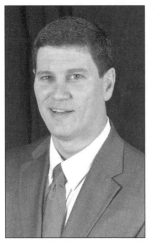

Thomas G. Guilliams Ph.D. earned his doctorate from the Medical College of Wisconsin (Milwaukee) where he studied molecular immunology in the Microbiology Department. Since 1996, he has spent his time studying the mechanisms and actions of natural-based therapies, and is an expert in the therapeutic uses of nutritional supplements. As the VP of Science and Regulatory Affairs for Ortho Molecular Products, he has developed a wide array of products and programs which allow clinicians to use nutritional supplements and lifestyle interventions as safe, evidence-based and effective tools for a variety of patients. Tom teaches at the University of Wisconsin School of Pharmacy, where he holds an appointment as a Clinical Instructor; at the University of Minnesota School of Pharmacy and is a faculty member of the Fellowship in Anti-aging Regenerative and Functional Medicine. He lives outside of Stevens Point, Wisconsin with his wife and 6 children.

To see Dr. Guilliams' other writings, go to The Point Institute—www.pointinstitute.org.

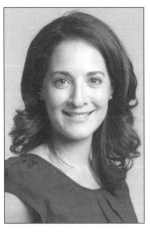

Roni Enten M.Sc. is a Certified Nutrition Specialist and a Licensed Dietitian-Nutritionist (LDN). She received her B.S.N. in Natural Health and Nutrition from Bastyr University and her M.Sc. in Nutrition Sciences from the Hebrew University of Jerusalem. Roni writes about nutrition and healthy lifestyle and also consults with adults and families of special needs children about nutrition and special diets, using a biomedical approach. Roni's writings have been published in books, peer-reviewed journals, magazines and blogs.